The complete set of books in
Creating Successful Dementia Care Settings
includes

Volume 1: **Understanding the Environment Through Aging Senses**
Volume 2: **Maximizing Cognitive and Functional Abilities**
Volume 3: **Minimizing Disruptive Behaviors**
Volume 4: **Enhancing Identity and Sense of Home**

Training videos for
Creating Successful Dementia Care Settings
include

Maximizing Cognitive and Functional Abilities (companion to Volume 2)
Minimizing Disruptive Behaviors (companion to Volume 3)
Enhancing Self and Sense of Home (companion to Volume 4)
(See ordering information at end of book.)

Creating Successful Dementia Care Settings

Developed by Margaret P. Calkins, M.Arch., Ph.D.

Volume 3
Minimizing Disruptive Behaviors

Volume Authors
Kristin Perez, OTR/L,
Mark A. Proffitt, M.Arch.,
and Margaret P. Calkins, M.Arch., Ph.D.

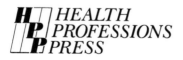
HEALTH
PROFESSIONS
PRESS

Baltimore • London • Winnipeg • Sydney

Health Professions Press, Inc.
Post Office Box 10624
Baltimore, Maryland 21285-0624

www.healthpropress.com

Typeset by Barton Matheson Willse & Worthington, Baltimore, Maryland.
Printed in the United States of America by Versa Press, Inc., East Peoria, Illinois.
Interior illustrations by David Fedan.

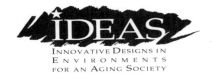

INNOVATIVE DESIGNS IN
E N V I R O N M E N T S
FOR AN AGING SOCIETY

Margaret P. Calkins, M.Arch., Ph.D., is president of I.D.E.A.S. (Innovative Designs
in Environments for an Aging Society), Inc., a consultation, education, and research
firm dedicated to exploring the therapeutic potential of the environment as it relates
to older adults who are frail and impaired. I.D.E.A.S., Inc., is based in Kirtland, Ohio.

The case examples in this book series are based on the authors' actual experiences. In
all instances, names and identifying details have been changed to protect confiden-
tiality.

Library of Congress Cataloging-in-Publication Data

Calkins, Margaret P.
    Creating successful dementia care settings / developed by Margaret P. Calkins.
      p.   cm.
    Includes bibliographical references and index.
    Contents: Vol. 1. Understanding the environment through aging senses—v. 2.
Maximizing cognitive and functional abilities—v. 3. Minimizing disruptive behaviors—v. 4. Enhancing identity and sense of home.
    ISBN 1-878812-72-6 (v. 1)—ISBN 1-878812-73-4 (v. 2)—ISBN 1-878812-74-2 (v.
3)—ISBN 1-878812-75-0 (v. 4)
    1. Dementia—Patients—Care. 2. Dementia—Patients—Long-term care. 3.
Health facilities—Administration. I. Title.

RC521.C35 2001
362.1′9683—dc21   2001039141

British Cataloguing in Publication Data are available from the British Library.

Series
Contents

Volume 2

Volume 3

Volume 4

About the Authors

Margaret P. Calkins, M.Arch., Ph.D., is President of I.D.E.A.S. Inc. (Innovative Designs in Environments for an Aging Society), a consultation, education, and research firm dedicated to exploring the therapeutic potential of the environment—social and organizational as well as physical—particularly as it relates to older adults who are frail and impaired. She is also Senior Fellow Emeritus of the Institute on Aging and Environment at the University of Wisconsin-Milwaukee.

Dr. Calkins holds degrees in both psychology and architecture. A member of several national organizations and panels that focus on issues of care for older adults with cognitive impairment, she speaks frequently at conferences nationally and internationally. She has published extensively, and her book *Design for Dementia: Planning Environments for the Elderly and the Confused* (National Health Publication, 1998) was the first comprehensive design guide for special care units for people with dementia.

Dr. Calkins is Director and a founding member of SAGE (Society for the Advancement of Gerontological Environments), and has been a juror for numerous design competitions.

Sherylyn H. Briller, Ph.D., is Assistant Professor of Anthropology at Wayne State University. She is a medical anthropologist who specializes in aging research. Dr. Briller received her master's and doctorate degrees and a graduate certificate in gerontology from Case Western Reserve University. She has been actively involved in the field of aging for more than a decade, both domestically and abroad. Her diverse career has included working as an activities coordinator in a skilled nursing facility, a program director at a community senior center, and a gerontological researcher in the United States of America and Asia. Her long-term care expertise includes philosophy/model of care, staff training, activity programming, and ethnic/cultural issues relating to aging. She has consulted, published, and given presentations to numerous audiences including policy makers, researchers, administrators, direct caregivers, and consumers.

John P. Marsden, M.Arch., Ph.D., is an assistant professor in the College of Design, Construction and Planning and a core faculty member of the Institute on Aging at the University of Florida. He holds degrees in architecture from Carnegie Mellon University, the University of Arizona, and the University of Michigan. Dr. Marsden has worked for several architecture firms, was an associate at I.D.E.A.S., Inc., and has consulted with designers and long-term care administrators. He is a frequent speaker at gerontology and environmental design conferences and served as a juror for the 1999 Best of Seniors' Housing Awards, sponsored by the National Council on Seniors' Housing, a division of the National Association of Home Builders.

Kristin Perez, OTR/L, received her bachelor's degree in gerontology from Bowling Green State University and a certificate in occupational therapy from Cleveland State University. Ms. Perez has experience in direct care, programming, management, and research in dementia care settings. She has assisted older adults in maximizing their level of independence and life satisfaction in assisted living, nursing facility, adult day services, and hospital settings. Ms. Perez has been actively involved in numerous research projects addressing dementia care practices and environments, including project management. She has also provided consultation to long-term care facilities regarding dementia care practices and environmental influences.

Mark A. Proffitt, M.Arch., is an architectural researcher with Dorsky Hodgson + Partners, an architectural firm that specializes in designs for older adults. His primary responsibilities include post-occupancy evaluations of completed projects and the programming protocol for the elderly design studio. He strongly believes that good design must build on research. Mr. Proffitt received his master's degree in architecture from the University of Wisconsin–Milwaukee, where he was a fellow with the Institute on Aging and Environment. After receiving his degree, he served as a facilities architect and manager for a developer of retirement communities. Mr. Proffitt has also co-authored a book on the creation and evaluation of an innovative health center and has spoken at several industry-related conferences.

Acknowledgments

Creative endeavors are nurtured to fruition by the ideas and efforts of myriad people at every step of a process. While the original conceptualization for the project was spearheaded by Maggie Calkins, with input from Jerry Weisman, this was very much a team project. All of the authors' talents and contributions were integral and critical to the evolution of the larger project from which these volumes are drawn. In addition, Eileen Lipstreuer, Chari Weber, and Rebecca Meehan deserve as much credit for their contributions to the project as the names that appear on the title pages of these volumes. The videos that accompany these volumes are a direct result of their industriousness. Thanks also to Jesse Epstein, of Cinecraft, and David Litz, the videographer, and to David Fedan for his charming illustrations.

Much of the project was funded by the National Institute on Aging (grant R44 AG12311) and enthusiastically supported and championed by Marcia Ory. We were also fortunate to have a team of nationally recognized experts whose input—both conceptual and practical—was invaluable. We extend our gratitude to Powell Lawton, Jerry Weisman, Phil Sloane, Joe Foley, Susan Gilster, Kitty Buckwalter, Jeanne Teresi, Doug Holmes, and Sheryl Zimmerman. Peter Whitehouse, Elisabeth Koss, Clive Gilmore, and Monte Levinson shared their keen intellect and significant insight with us as we started this project. During the most stressful periods of the project, Cassie and Ted always seemed to come to our rescue.

We would like to thank the numerous individuals whose publications and conference presentations enriched our understanding of the complex nature of dementia, and provided myriad ideas for creative solutions to difficult challenges. We also appreciate the endless hours of listening and thoughtful contributions of the many family, friends, and colleagues who helped out in so many ways as the project evolved over 4 years. To the numerous facility staff and administrators who listened to, read, questioned, and critiqued our efforts and dialogued with us about them, it was for you that we embarked on this voyage. We are pleased to share what we have learned with you.

Preface

All too often, we see well-intentioned caregivers unnecessarily limit or downplay the potential remaining abilities of the older adults with dementia for whom they care. Caregivers seem to assume that because a person has dementia, every behavior and every expression of anxiety, fear, or anger is a direct consequence of the dementing illness. And, because dementia impairs care recipients' cognitive abilities, many caregivers believe that they have the right and the responsibility to make all decisions for those they care for.

It has been the authors' experience that the factors that affect the behavior of residents with dementia are complex. Our approach to understanding their behavior focuses on the person, on his or her typical needs and desires, on the limitations imposed by age-related changes, and on the effects of aspects of the environment.

Our fundamental philosophy is that we must first consider those in our care as people, who have many of the same needs, desires, and wishes as anyone else. To lose the ability to make decisions that affect virtually every aspect of living is devastating. To have that ability further eroded by care providers and care settings that eliminate almost every opportunity for choice and control is unacceptable.

It is the authors' hope that in using the information contained within *Creating Successful Dementia Care Settings*, facilities will create meaningful care settings by educating and sensitizing staff and by making full use of the environmental resources available to them.

User's Guide

The authors' goal in writing this four-volume series was to create an easy-to-use reference to help care providers understand and more appropriately manage, through the environment, the broad array of behaviors and changing abilities that occur with dementia. One must first recognize the importance of accommodating the basic needs of all people, and then one must consider that most people with dementia are older and, therefore, experience the world through sensory modalities that are changing or that have been altered by aging. Vision, hearing, touch, taste, and smell all change with age, and sensory changes often affect behavior. For example, it may not be dementia but simply poor vision that hinders a person's ability to read signs or an activity calendar. Volume 1, *Understanding the Environment Through Aging Senses* helps caregivers to be more sensitive to how these sensory changes can affect a person's basic functioning.

Only after the needs of the resident as a person like anyone else and as an older person with changing sensory experiences have been acknowledged can one consider the unique needs of the individual as an older person with dementia. There is no denying that the neuropathological changes that occur in the brain of a person with dementia affect his or her ability to perceive, make sense of, and operate effectively in the surrounding environment. Basic tasks, such as dressing and eating, that once were easy become increasingly difficult. The inability to interpret what someone is saying, to identify faces or objects, or to understand his or her current location can easily lead to fear and resistance to care. Volumes 2 and 3, *Maximizing Cognitive and Functional Abilities* and *Minimizing Disruptive Behaviors*, respectively, focus on these issues.

Enhancing Identity and Sense of Home, Volume 4, addresses issues that are primarily related to basic human needs such as privacy, autonomy, identity, and personal space. Much of the information is appropriate not only for people with dementia but also for cognitively alert individuals in long-term care settings.

The more that you, as a caregiver, understand all of the factors that affect the person or people whose care is entrusted to you, the better able you are to see the world as they do. Thus, the beginning of each chapter in all of the volumes presents the individual topic from the residents' perspective, including contributing factors and influences on specific behaviors or issues. In addition, these sections offer ideas for assessing problems and implementing interventions. This level of information is particularly useful for staff members who manage and/or train direct care staff. The authors hope that this information will broaden staff's knowledge on the topic and that they will pass the information along to others who care for residents.

The residents' perspective section is followed by "What Staff Can Do," which provides information on social interactions between staff and residents and ideas for structured and spontaneous activities on the unit. Some interventions focus on teaching direct care staff to take a different approach to particular situations, whereas other interventions are provided for staff who plan structured activities and programs.

The third main section of each chapter, "What the Environment Can Do," offers suggestions for modifications or changes that can be made to the physical environment so that your facility becomes more supportive of the residents, particularly those with dementia. Many of the suggested changes cost nothing and involve only a different use of the environment or a small modification using materials you probably already have on hand. Other changes are low in cost, requiring the purchase of a few additional products or materials. Finally, if your facility is able to upgrade or replace some of its furnishings or equipment, we have provided practical advice in "What the Environment Can Do" on what to consider when purchasing a product. Many of the modifications suggested in this section explain how these modifications benefit the residents and the staff who care for them.

The final section of each chapter, "Where to Find Products," lists specific manufacturers and distributors of the products mentioned in the text. There is some repetition in these sections across the four volumes so that you do not have to refer to a separate volume for the information. Many of the manufacturers and catalogs also carry more products than those highlighted in our lists. This section is followed by a summary sheet, which boils down the chapter text into an easy-to-remember, quick overview. We have also provided an area for you to make notes about your own staff and facility. Managerial staff may wish to use the summary sheets as handouts to accompany direct care staff training, or to post them by the time clock or nurses' station or include them in staff's pay envelopes. All staff, including business office, social services, dietary, and housekeeping, may appreciate this quick overview of issues because they likely interact with residents daily.

At the conclusion of each volume, a detailed bibliography and suggested readings help you learn more about issues in the individual volumes. The Behavior Tracking Form and Sensory Stimulation Assessment appendixes appear at the end of Volume 3. Staff can use these forms to examine the occurrence of behaviors and aspects of the environment more closely. Each blank form is accompanied by explanatory information and a sample completed form. Volume 4 includes three appendixes, all designed to help residents feel more at home in the facility and to protect their safety.

In addition to the four volumes, there are three videotapes that relate to Volumes 2–4. They were designed to be staff education resources and provide an additional way of helping all staff learn how to create successful dementia care settings (see ordering information at the end of each volume).

We at I.D.E.A.S., Inc., wish you success in developing a high-quality environment for caregiving. It is our hope that facilities will use this information to create meaningful dementia care settings by educating and sensitizing staff. If you are having a hard time determining which aspects of your care setting most need to be changed or modified, we hope that you will contact us directly (440-256-1880 or info@IDEASconsultingInc.com).

1

What Is Disruptive Behavior?

It is not uncommon to see individuals with dementia exhibiting behaviors that are disruptive to the people around them. In long-term care settings these behaviors can be frustrating for staff, other residents, visitors, and even the residents who are exhibiting the behaviors. This volume highlights some of the behaviors that are commonly seen, including

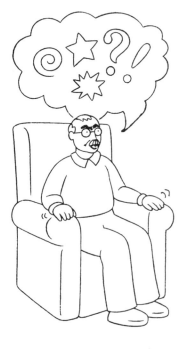

- Wandering
- Attempting to leave
- Rummaging and hoarding
- Combative behaviors
- Socially inappropriate behaviors

The term *wandering* sometimes is used in the literature to describe a wide range of behaviors. For example, attempts to leave a facility or rummaging in another resident's room sometimes are considered a part of wandering. Although these behaviors often are related (e.g., a resident wanders into another resident's room and then starts to rummage), the causes for these behaviors and the effects and implications that they have can vary significantly. Therefore, wandering and rummaging are addressed individually. For the purposes of this volume, *wandering* is defined as a form of walking in which a person either does not have an apparent goal or is in search of someone or something that is unattainable. This definition is based on other descriptions of wandering in the literature.

Combative behavior is another term that has been defined in different ways in the literature. In addition, other terms such as *aggressive behaviors*, *agitation*, and *resistance to care* commonly are used to describe such behavior.

Therefore, for the purposes of this volume, the following definitions have been developed for various combative behaviors:

- *Physical combativeness* refers to negative physical behaviors that occur in response to specific staff–resident or resident–resident interactions (e.g., a resident strikes out at a staff member who is trying to feed him or her).
- *Verbal combativeness* refers to negative verbal outbursts in response to specific staff–resident or resident–resident interactions (e.g., a resident yells at a staff member who is undressing him or her).
- *Aggressive behavior* is initiated by the resident and is not exhibited as an obvious response to a specific interpersonal interaction. Aggressive behaviors can be physical or verbal (e.g., a resident strikes someone with no apparent provocation).

Because combative behaviors almost always are exhibited in response to something, truly aggressive behaviors, as defined here, occur infrequently. Therefore, throughout this volume, the term *combative,* which refers to both physical and verbal behaviors, is used.

Chapter 6 of this volume addresses three different types of behaviors that often are viewed as socially inappropriate. The first behavior that is addressed is disruptive vocalizations such as calling out and moaning. Next, sexual behaviors are addressed. This section of Chapter 6 addresses issues of residents' sexuality, including relationships with others, masturbation, and disrobing in public. Some of these behaviors are not inherently inappropriate (e.g., wanting to have an intimate relationship with someone); however, for reasons such as the presence of dementia, such relationships may not be possible in a resident's situation. Finally, repetitive behaviors, including both movements and vocalizations, are addressed. Throughout the other chapters of this volume, references are made to the issues that are examined in the following sections of this chapter (e.g., tracking behaviors). The reader is encouraged to refer to this text when planning to implement a process or an intervention.

PAST RESPONSES TO DISRUPTIVE BEHAVIORS

Disruptive behaviors are not a new problem in long-term care facilities, but the interventions to respond to them are evolving. For many years, residents who engaged in disruptive behaviors were restrained, either physically or with psychotropic medications. As more has been learned about Alzheimer's disease and related disorders, and with the passage of the Omnibus Budget Reconciliation Act of 1987 (PL 100-203), this practice is becoming less common. The Resident's Rights section of this law states that residents of long-term care facilities have the right to be free from physical and chemical restraints and that restraints may not be used for discipline or staff's convenience. Restraints may be used only 1) to ensure the physical safety of the resident or other residents and 2) when the resident's physician has written an order that specifies the duration for and circumstances under which a restraint can be used.

Physical restraints should not be used as an intervention for residents engaged in combative behavior, unless a sincere concern for physical harm exists. In fact, restraining these residents is likely to make them even more combative and distressed. Ryden et al. (1999) found that the use of restraints, the use of antipsychotic medications, and placement on a secure unit all were significantly related to higher levels of physical aggression. These authors did not explore why living on a secure unit increased aggression; however, this behavior likely was related to feelings of confinement and loss of control. (Chapter 3 discusses how these feelings can be minimized when residents have access to a secure outdoor area.) There are some situations and conditions, such as severe paranoia or hallucinations, in which psychotropic medications may be an appropriate intervention. They should be used only as a last resort, after other interventions have been tried.

Regulations regarding restraints have been in effect since the early 1990s. In that time, most long-term care facilities have made significant strides to reduce the use of restraints and implement alternative interventions. Staff have begun to learn about how the negative side effects that are associated with restraints often outweigh any benefits. Numerous publications have highlighted restraint reduction success stories. For example, Johnson (1995), a former director of nursing, described how her facility became restraint-free in less than a year. Although the inappropriate use of restraints has decreased significantly, it still exists in many facilities. In fact, restraint use remains one of the 10 most frequent violations in surveys of long-term care facilities (16.3% of U.S. facilities; Bua, 1997).

These findings suggest that many long-term care staff are not aware of enough appropriate and successful alternative interventions. This volume and the others in this series attempt to educate long-term care staff about new ways to approach behavior management and to empower them to try new interventions. This volume looks at why residents may engage in certain behaviors, examines how problematic the behaviors truly are, and provides ideas about how to either prevent or respond to such behaviors.

WHY DO THESE BEHAVIORS OCCUR?

Although disruptive behaviors are observed frequently in residents with dementia, they usually are not merely the result of the dementing illness. In almost all cases, something triggers the behavior. The challenge for staff is to identify the trigger. In some cases, the residents' words or actions make the cause of the behavior fairly obvious. For example, a resident who is trying to leave the unit may tell you that he or she needs to go home. Although going home may not be possible or realistic, the resident has expressed a normal and understandable reason for wanting to leave. Likewise, when a resident reacts combatively after repeatedly saying that he or she does not want a bath, it is fairly easy to understand that the resident is reacting in this manner because someone is trying to get him or her to do something that he or she does not want to do. At other times, staff may not know what triggered a behavior. In either case, staff not only need to figure out what caused the behavior but also to determine how to prevent behaviors that create stressful situations for themselves and the residents and how to respond to disruptive behaviors when they do occur. The following sections discuss some concepts that can be applied to a variety of behaviors and situations.

Agenda Behavior Approach

The belief that there is almost always some cause behind a behavior is supported by a concept referred to as the *agenda behavior approach,* which was developed by three nurse researchers (Rader, Doan, & Schwab, 1985). Rader and colleagues defined agenda behaviors as "the verbal and nonverbal planning and actions that the cognitively impaired persons use in an attempt to fulfill their felt social, emotional and physical needs" (p. 196). This approach indicates that it is important to determine why a resident is doing something before staff try to change that behavior. Rader et al. suggested that behaviors such as wandering, attempting to leave, and aggression are often the result of feelings of loneliness and separation. Having one's agenda prevented or disrupted can lead to frustration and agitation. Thus, a main goal of this approach is to enable each resident to carry out his or her agenda behavior to the greatest extent possible. For example, if a resident wants to leave, then he or she should be allowed to do so. If the facility does not have a secure courtyard that the resident could go to on his or her own, then a staff member should accompany the resident. Using this approach, the staff member could ask the resident for permission to accompany him or her. Then, after walking a few minutes, the resident may initiate returning to the building or be receptive to the staff member's suggesting that they go back inside. Rader et al.

found that when residents were allowed to carry out their agenda, disruptive behavior recurred less frequently.

This approach is useful for addressing many disruptive behaviors and is referred to throughout this volume. Initially, administrators may believe that they simply do not have enough staff and/or enough staff time to implement this approach. However, although the agenda behavior approach does require additional staff time during the episode, it can save staff time in dealing with disruptive behaviors when they are occurring less often. In addition, with appropriate training, volunteers can help implement this approach. If implementing this approach at your facility would be helpful but you have concerns as to how administrators will respond, the original article by Rader et al. (1985) presents a strong case for how this approach could benefit the residents and staff of the facility.

Using a Behavior Tracking Process

The agenda behavior approach addresses the fact that residents have reasons for their behaviors and that allowing a behavior can help fulfill a personal need. In many cases this approach is an appropriate intervention. Some behaviors, such as combativeness, should be prevented, however. Likewise, understanding why residents engage in particular disruptive behaviors may help to determine alternative methods or activities for fulfilling their needs or desires. For example, when a resident expresses a desire to go home to his or her family, assisting the resident to telephone a family member helps to fulfill his or her need to be with family in a more feasible manner. Of course, residents with dementia cannot always tell you why they act in a particular manner. Therefore, staff need to become adept at observing residents' actions and body language as well as what else is happening in the environment at the time. A behavior tracking process can be used to help staff examine behaviors that are disruptive or troubling. The behavior tracking process involves the following six steps:

1. *Define the Issue:* Determine what behavior(s) you want to track and for which resident(s). If the facility has a number of residents who are combative during personal care, then you may want to track combative behaviors for all residents. Alternatively, a resident may engage in a number of disruptive behaviors, and you may wish to track all of the behaviors in which he or she engages.

2. *Track the Behavior:* Tracking a resident's behavior allows you to look for patterns and may help you to determine what influences the behavior (see Appendix A). Tracking involves recording some basic information each time a behavior occurs. The 5 Ws—who, what

(e.g., what behavior), where, when, and why—are useful for this process (see also Volume 2 for more information on the 5 Ws). For the purpose of tracking resident behavior, the 5 Ws are defined as

- Who (name of the resident) exhibited the behavior?
- What was the resident doing, and what was happening on the unit?
- When did the behavior occur?
- Where did the behavior occur?
- Why do you think the resident behaved this way?

With regard to the last of the 5 Ws, the reason why a resident acted in a particular way may not be evident, but it is helpful if staff record anything that they think may have caused the behavior. A Behavior Tracking Form is provided in Appendix A. This form can be used in tracking resident behavior, or you may wish to develop your own. Appendix A also includes an example with some sample entries to give you an idea as to how to fill out the form.

The tracking process does not have to take much staff time; however, it is important for all staff who work on the unit to be aware of it. The staff member initiating the behavior tracking should meet with staff members from all shifts to explain to them the purpose of the tracking process and how the findings may help them better work with the resident. It is important to emphasize that this tracking may lead to response strategies that are better suited to the resident(s), and therefore more effective. This, in turn, likely will mean less time involvement and frustration on the part of staff.

3. *Learn the Resident's History:* Another important part of determining patterns and influences on behavior is to speak to the individuals who are most familiar with the resident, such as family members. For example, ask the family whether the resident who spends a lot of time wandering around the facility wandered while he or she was still living at home. If so, how did they respond to it? Did their response work? Staff also should ask the family whether the person was physically active throughout his or her life. It is likely that someone who always was active feels a need to continue to be active. It is also important to talk to the direct care staff who work with residents. It is possible that a staff member has found a strategy that works but has not shared it with staff from other shifts. (See the social and residential history forms in Appendix A in Volume 4 to create a permanent document for staff to refer to.)

4. *Develop Intervention Strategies:* Once you begin to understand some of the resident's reasons for a behavior and any patterns he or she may exhibit, you can begin to brainstorm possible intervention strategies.
5. *Select a Strategy and Implement It:* Determine which strategy you think will work best for each resident. Inform staff of your decision, and begin to implement it.
6. *Reevaluate the Resident's Behavior:* If you do not see the desired results, then begin the process again.

Implementing a behavior tracking process requires some additional staff training, or at least a brief meeting with the staff of each shift to explain the process to them. When discussing the tracking process with staff, the key elements to touch on include the behavior(s) for which they should look, where the tracking form will be kept, what kind of information you would like staff to record, and the time frame for the tracking process. Let staff know that, after the information is collected, you will use the information to try to identify interventions specific to each resident exhibiting the behavior. It is helpful to brainstorm these interventions with at least some of the direct care staff. Emphasize how finding effective interventions for residents' disruptive behaviors will make their jobs easier and more satisfying.

The tracking process is most beneficial to residents and staff if a staff training session is conducted that not only explains how to implement the tracking process but also teaches staff about the various influences for specific disruptive behaviors. Once they have a better understanding of the types of factors that can influence resident behavior, they may find it easier to think of their own interventions for these behaviors or of ways to interact differently with residents. In addition, this knowledge enables staff to be more specific in the information they record on the tracking forms.

The Behavior Tracking Form is designed to be completed for an individual disruptive behavior (e.g., leaving the unit). Therefore, the form may be used for multiple residents; however, if the behavior is particularly frequent for a specific resident, then you may want to consider creating a form just for him or her. Although you may wish to track a number of behaviors on your unit, it is best to focus on only one or two at a time. This enables direct care staff to record occurrences as accurately as possible without feeling that they are spending too much time doing so.

In this volume, the introductory sections of each chapter describe the disruptive behaviors that residents engage in and potential causes of and influences on these behaviors. "What Staff Can Do" and "What the Environment Can Do" offer programmatic and environmental interventions for either preventing or responding to these behaviors.

2
Wandering

There is no doubt that residents with dementia who wander pose a challenge to all levels of staff in long-term care settings. Wandering is a behavior that has been widely studied, with different researchers defining it differently. Therefore, this section first defines wandering for the purposes of this volume. Next, there is a discussion of various topics related to wandering, such as

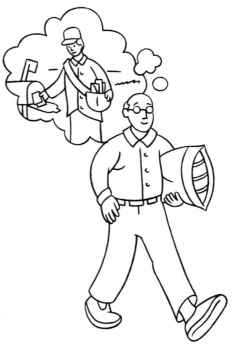

- What can lead to wandering behaviors
- Determination of the causes of wandering
- What differentiates wanderers from nonwanderers

Finally, "What Staff Can Do" and "What the Environment Can Do" offer some strategies that can be used to help minimize wandering.

WHAT IS WANDERING?

Wandering is a form of walking in which a person either does not have an apparent goal, or is in search of someone or something that is currently unattainable. This definition is built on other descriptions of wandering from the literature that looked at different issues, such as whether the wanderer had a

Table 2.1.   What is wandering?

	Goal oriented (1)	Non-goal oriented (2)
Direct path (a)	Walking to desired location Exercise (1a)	Pacing Excessive walking (2a)
Non-direct path (b)	Has a goal, but is disoriented to current space/activity Looking for unattainable place or person Forgetting where desired location is (1b)	Aimless wandering Restless walking (2b)

According to the text definition of wandering, the shaded boxes (1b, 2a, 2b) are considered "wandering."

goal or the wanderer's travel pattern. Table 2.1 and the following description help illustrate this definition of wandering in more detail.

Table 2.1 suggests that people either have a goal (1), which may or may not be attainable or realistic, or do not have a goal/destination in mind (2). Likewise, they walk either in a direct path (a) or in a nondirect path (b). Therefore, when residents have a goal, such as going from the bedroom to the dining room, and take a direct path to that goal, this is not wandering (1a). If they cannot find the dining room and get lost, then they have a goal but follow a nondirect path, and this is considered wandering (1b). If a resident is looking for his or her mother or childhood home, which are not attainable in the current situation (there is no direct path to take to the goal), then this is also wandering (1b). Someone who is moving around with no goal also is considered to be wandering (2a and 2b).

Wandering in and of itself is not disruptive; it is the behaviors that are associated with wandering that cause problems. These associated behaviors include excessive walking, attempting to leave the unit/facility, rummaging, and invading other residents' personal space and territory. Once these behaviors are separated from wandering, staff can reassess whether wandering truly is a problem on the unit.

Attempting to leave and rummaging in others' belongings are different behaviors from wandering and thus are addressed in separate chapters of this volume. However, because residents' reasons for walking excessively are often similar to those for wandering, excessive walking is included within this chapter. Excessive walking ((2a) in Table 2.1) is another form of movement that is commonly seen in long-term care settings. This behavior could be seen as wandering taken to the extreme because residents who exhibit this behavior usually spend the majority of their waking time walking. Excessive walking often is seen as more problematic than wandering because it sometimes results in negative effects such as weight loss, fatigue, dehydration, and foot problems. Interventions for excessive walking are listed at the ends of "What Staff Can Do" and "What the Environment Can Do."

MOTIVATORS FOR WANDERING

Wandering, as well as other disruptive behaviors, often has a goal or purpose. These goals or purposes are often referred to as agenda behaviors because they are aimed at addressing a purpose (Rader et al., 1985). At other times, residents may wander without a conscious reason. Some residents with dementia may wander in response to stress, expressing their agitation through pacing or restless walking. For others, wandering may stem from an inability to make sense of the environment. Researchers have identified a number of psychosocial factors that can influence wandering behavior (Anthony, 1991; Martino-Saltzman, Blasch, Morris, & Wynn McNeal, 1991). These factors are listed in Table 2.2, with examples for each.

Another characteristic of wanderers is that their cognitive impairments often differ from those of nonwanderers. Wanderers are more likely to have cognitive impairments that are irreversible. Wanderers also are more likely to have impaired language skills (Algase, 1992b). Before they developed cognitive impairment, wanderers often were more social than nonwanderers. However, once cognitive impairment began, wanderers were found to spend more time alone than nonwanderers (Algase, 1992b). As more is learned about the causes and influences of wandering behavior and the characteristics of wanderers, it becomes easy to see how wandering could be a coping mechanism for some residents. For example,

Dorothy was always involved in numerous organizations and clubs. Increasing cognitive impairments caused a decline in Dorothy's social and language skills and led to her move to a long-term care facility. These changes combined to prevent Dorothy from doing the things that once kept her busy. She does not know (or recognize) many of the residents or staff on

her unit, nor is she sure of how to interact with them. Conse-
quently, she spends a lot of time wandering around the unit.
Wandering takes the place of the social activities she was used
to doing.

PAST RESPONSES TO WANDERING

In the past, long-term care facility residents who wandered often were physically or chemically restrained. Fortunately, reliance on restraints has decreased since the passage of the Omnibus Budget Reconciliation Act of 1987.
The guidelines in this act state that residents with behavior problems also
should exhibit psychotic symptoms or be a danger to themselves or others before neuroleptic medication is prescribed. In addition, a great deal of attention has been given to the negative effects of restraints. Use of restraints has
been associated with increased agitation, incontinence, and injury and decreased physical activity. Furthermore, physical restraints do little to reduce

Table 2.2.   Psychosocial factors that influence wandering

Psychosocial factors	Example
A need for security	A resident may be wandering in search of someone or something familiar.
Previous work roles	A resident may have had a profession that involved walking, such as mail delivery.
Impaired recent and remote memory	Memory impairments may cause a resident to forget where he or she is, what is happening, or what he or she did an hour ago and so forth, causing the resident to wander in search of something or someone he or she recognizes.
Orientation (or disorientation) to time and place	A resident may not be able to find a specific thing or place for which he or she is looking, such as a childhood home or deceased spouse.
Lifelong method of coping with stress	Throughout life, a resident may have taken a walk when under stress.
Diminished ability to make appropriate responses in conversation	Frustration over not being able to follow conversation may lead a resident to physically avoid conversation when possible.

fall-related injuries. One study found that psychotropic medications have little effect on behaviors such as agitation, and sometimes they actually increased wandering (Matteson & Linton, 1996). Although the use of many types of restraints has decreased significantly, it is important to remember that there are subtle forms of restraint, such as placing residents in recliners or beanbag chairs, that still have the same negative consequences.

STRATEGIES TO ADDRESS WANDERING

Most long-term care facilities have residents who wander. The exception to this is facilities that carefully plan their programs with the interests, personal history, and abilities of each resident in mind. This discussion offers some general approaches for responding to wandering behavior and turning an often-challenging situation into a pleasant one. "What Staff Can Do" and "What the Environment Can Do" offer specific recommendations to consider.

A number of alternative strategies can be used to address wandering behaviors. It is important for staff to determine what influences each wandering resident. If wandering is a new problem for a particular resident, then medical staff should conduct an evaluation to identify potential problems with medications or other changes in health status. Once health and medication issues have been addressed, it is important to develop a strategy for responding to wandering. The behavior tracking process described in Chapter 1 of this volume can be helpful in this regard. Possible intervention strategies for wandering include

- Allowing the wandering to continue
- Attempting to stop or redirect the wandering
- Addressing the wandering as an agenda behavior

The strategy of redirecting often is used when what a resident is doing, or is about to do, is seen as inappropriate or undesirable by staff, and they therefore try to prevent it by directing the resident to some other location or activity. Redirection can be done in a number of ways, ranging from a staff member redirecting a resident to a different area or activity to simply turning him or her away from a door or a particular area (see Figure 2.1).

Use of redirection for wandering behaviors is most successful when it involves something the resident can relate to or addresses one of the factors that influences his or her wandering. For instance, when Dorothy (from the previous example) wanders, she seems to always be in search of her children.

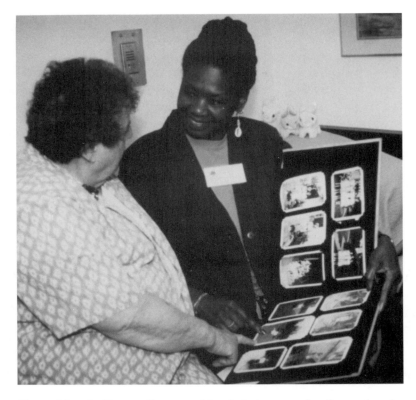

Figure 2.1.   Staff can redirect a resident's desire to see family members by providing the person with a family photo album.

One strategy that may reassure Dorothy is to ask her children to put together a small album of pictures of them. Then, when she is looking for them, staff could direct her to the album. Although this intervention is no substitute for actually seeing her children, seeing the pictures may bring back happy memories and help Dorothy to feel closer to them. Likewise, if Fred tends to wander a lot because he seems to need to stay busy, an appropriate strategy for him may be to involve him in an activity such as folding towels. This not only keeps Fred busy and therefore not wandering, but also gives him a feeling of usefulness.

The agenda behavior approach described in Chapter 1 is another recommended intervention (Rader et al., 1985). In essence, the agenda behavior approach suggests that people do things for a reason. Thus it is important to attempt to figure out *why* the resident is doing something before trying to change that behavior. Agenda behaviors include wandering, exiting, and ag-

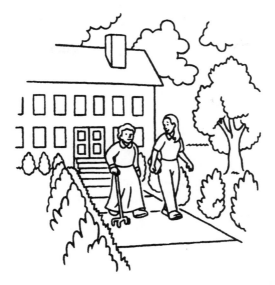

Figure 2.2. Following the agenda behavior approach may mean taking a walk with a resident who wants to be outside.

gression. A main goal of this approach is to enable the resident to carry out his or her agenda behavior (see Figure 2.2).

WHAT STAFF CAN DO

Those who have worked for a while in long-term care settings know that there are always some residents who spend a lot of time wandering. Presumably, this wandering can be diminished if residents spend more time participating in planned activities and programs. The challenge is finding activities and programs that interest residents and keep their attention. At one time or another, most staff have seen residents get up and leave an ongoing program. Although this can be frustrating and unfortunately sometimes sets off a chain reaction of resident departures, there is no reason to give up on these residents. That particular activity may not have held their interest, but they may well benefit from or enjoy other social activities and interactions.

This section provides some ideas and suggestions for programming for residents who are prone to wander. The terms *programming* and *activities* refer not only to structured and planned activities but also to everything in which residents engage over the course of the day. This section also addresses orientation because residents' wandering sometimes occurs as a result of their disorientation.

Inhibitors to Social Involvement

Research has found that, in general, wanderers with cognitive impairment tended to be more social prior to experiencing cognitive impairment than were wanderers without cognitive impairment (Algase, 1992b; Monsour & Robb, 1982). It has been suggested that wandering sometimes may be a substitute for social interaction. Thus, wandering residents may be searching for something to do but lack the ability to initiate an activity or even a conversation on their own. Researchers also have found that wanderers with dementia often have greater impairment of their language skills than do residents with dementia who do not wander (Algase, 1992b). Keeping this in mind, it is important that staff offer some programs and activities that do not require a great deal of conversation or rely on complex directions.

Also, wandering sometimes may be a resident's way of alleviating feelings of anxiety. Thus, it is important that activities in which wanderers participate do not cause or add to any feelings of anxiety. This is least likely to happen when activities are planned that meet the participating residents' levels of physical and cognitive functioning. When residents feel both interest in the current activity and the ability to succeed at it, they experience feelings of accomplishment and self-worth instead of anxiety.

Promoting Social Involvement

Activities from the Past

The cognitive impairments of residents with dementia make it more difficult for them to learn new activities. The most successful activities for residents to do independently likely will be ones that relate to familiar things that they are used to doing. Staff should talk to the residents, their family and friends, or both about the residents' interests. Once interests are identified, staff should try to develop specific programs and activities that address these interests.

Residents can engage in some activities without much staff intervention. An extremely successful intervention that involved an activity from residents' past was the creation of a "bowling alley" in the hallway of a Wisconsin nursing facility (Figure 2.3). The alley consisted of heavy-duty tape placed on the floor of a little-used hallway on the unit. The pins and a heavy rubber ball were left out all the time. The residents eventually formed leagues to structure

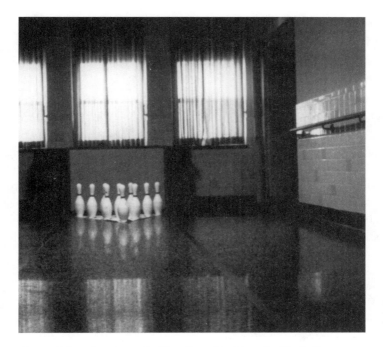

Figure 2.3. Creation of a "bowling alley" in a facility hallway provides residents with an activity with which most are familiar.

their playing (men in the morning, women in the afternoon, and mixed leagues in the evenings). These residents were lower functioning, with few verbal or physical capabilities and short attention spans. However, bowling is so popular in Wisconsin that almost every resident was capable of participating in the sport at some level. It was a skill they had not lost.

The first task in developing activities from the past is to discover what residents enjoyed doing throughout their lives. Staff should talk with the residents and their families about activities they enjoyed and then determine how they can be incorporated into the unit so that residents can engage in these activities with little or no staff intervention required. Suggestions include folding laundry (shirts for higher functioning intact residents, and towels and napkins for lower functioning residents), putting golf balls, or sorting socks. If the weather is nice, laundry can be hung outside if clotheslines are available. Men might enjoy painting, washing cars, raking leaves, and sanding wood. Other possible regional activities might be porch sitting, going to a barber or beauty shop for gossip, eating at a diner, or having potluck suppers or a Friday night fish fry. Many excellent resources are available on activity programming for residents with dementia (see "Where to Find Products" at the end of the chapter and the Bibliography at the end of the book for sources).

Structured Exercise in Place of Wandering

Some residents may have led active and busy lives before their cognitive and physical skills became impaired by dementia. Therefore, they may not be used to the more sedentary or passive lifestyle found in many long-term care settings. Wandering may be simply an attempt to stay active. If there is concern about residents' unmonitored wandering, then staff should consider providing more structured walking and exercise programs for these residents. Some facilities have started walking clubs and kept track of the distance that residents travel. Such programs can be a healthy way of allowing residents the freedom to move around and be active while giving the facility the reassurance that the wandering residents are supervised. The more involved wandering residents are with structured activities and programs, the less time they will have to wander around the facility.

Here are some helpful hints for successful programming for wanderers:

- Hold activities and programs in places where there are few distractions.
- Plan activities that meet the participating residents' levels of functioning (physical and cognitive).
- Encourage residents who are prone to wander to participate in any exercise programs that are offered.
- Make time for staff or a volunteer to be able to walk along with residents at times when they are wandering. These individuals may be lonely and might really benefit from spending some one-to-one time with someone. We all have a basic need for social contact, even if we can no longer communicate this to others. Wanderers often have feelings of loneliness and isolation, and these can be alleviated when staff

make an effort to connect with particular residents and form a relationship with them.

- Try to engage residents in an activity at the time of shift change because all of the related activity and noise may produce wandering behavior. Likewise, if behavior tracking records indicate other times when wandering is more prevalent or particularly disruptive, then try to design programs that will interest these residents at those times.
- Ask staff who work on the unit (nurses and certified nursing assistants) about the interests of the residents if you do not regularly work on the unit. The more activities you are able to offer residents that interest them, the greater your ability to reduce wandering.

Orientation

Residents with dementia may have trouble being oriented to their environment. Two methods of intervention that assist in orientation—reality orientation and use of cues—are particularly relevant for dealing with wandering behavior. (Additional information on this topic can be found in Volume 2, Chapter 2.)

Reality Orientation

Orientation, in general, refers to a person's awareness of his or her current situation, including an awareness and understanding of time, place, people, and what is happening. Residents with dementia often are confused about some of these things. Reality orientation is the practice of giving correct information to a resident who is confused about his or her current situation. An example of using reality orientation is telling a resident that her husband is deceased when she talks about him coming to visit. The advisability of orienting a resident to the present is a debatable topic. In general, great care should be taken when using traditional reality orientation with residents with dementia.

Some residents with mild to moderate cognitive impairments may ask staff for orientation cues (e.g., What day is today? Where are we?); in this case it is usually best to give them accurate information. However, it is probably not effective to try to train residents to remember facts such as date, season, and names. As cognitive impairment increases, reality orientation sometimes does more damage than good. Telling residents with more severe impairment something other than what they believe to be true may only frighten or upset them.

Mrs. Janikowski sometimes wanders around the facility saying that her husband is coming soon, but you know he has been deceased for 5 years. This is a sign that Mrs. Janikowski is dis-oriented to time and place (the current year and where she is). Telling Mrs. Janikowski that her husband is dead likely will be very upsetting to her because she obviously has "forgot-ten" this fact, and upsetting her could promote disruptive behav-iors (e.g., agitation, aggression, attempts to leave to find him). However, Mrs. Janikowski's talking about her husband may be a sign that she misses him and needs to feel close to him.

When staff encounter such a situation, they must think carefully before de-ciding how to respond. In this example, an alternative response could be to ask Mrs. Janikowski about her husband. Talking to you about him may be com-forting to her. It is possible that during the discussion she will come to the realiza-tion on her own that he has died and therefore will not be coming to visit her.

Using Cues to Help Orient Residents

Another form of orienta-tion that can be effective is providing physical and so-cial cues to the current activ-ity. For example, if the next activity is a coffee klatch, then staff can begin brewing coffee beforehand. This way, when a resi-dent enters the room or is directed there by staff, he or she will be able to asso-ciate the aroma of the coffee with what is going on. Likewise, an exercise ac-tivity could always start with the same exercise song.

Excessive Walking

Some residents walk regardless of what staff try to do. When carried to the ex-treme, this behavior is referred to as *excessive walking*. Staff may want or need to encourage these residents to rest periodically to avoid exhaustion. When a resident is being encouraged to rest, be sure to provide something of interest to touch or look at. By distracting the resident, you may be able to encourage longer periods of rest. Whatever is provided must be of interest to the resident. Books related to previous hobbies or texturally interesting objects may work best.

Music played through headphones may provide a calming influence on a resident whose wandering is caused by agitation. Headphones are preferred because the music is then heard without outside distractions, and it will not disturb other residents. If nutrition is an issue for residents who are constantly in motion, then consider providing finger foods that can be eaten easily "on the run" (Zgola & Bordillon, 2001).

WHAT THE ENVIRONMENT CAN DO

Some facilities view wandering as an inevitable consequence of dementia, and therefore do not believe that they need to develop an intervention unless the wandering is disruptive to other residents. Others think the term *wandering* is degrading and consider that residents are simply walking. The authors' position is somewhere in between. Wandering is not necessarily a problem to be corrected; however, a unit that has many residents who spend a great deal of time simply walking around probably is not providing enough or appropriate opportunities for residents to engage in social interaction. "What Staff Can Do" offers ideas for increasing social interaction. This section shares ideas on how the physical environment can be modified to promote social interaction. It also addresses adapting the environment to help orient residents who may be wandering in search of something or someplace and to deter residents from wandering into undesirable areas or other residents' bedrooms. Finally, this section discusses interventions for residents who walk excessively.

Promoting Social Interaction and Diversion

Seating Arrangements

Furniture arrangements either can foster more social interaction or can hinder this behavior. A great deal of communication is seen and not heard. For example, hand gestures and facial expressions often reinforce spoken communication. Therefore, furniture arrangements that promote face-to-face viewing help residents to communicate more effectively with one another. When furniture is lined up side by side (usually against the walls), it is more difficult for residents to engage in conversation. Chairs that are placed at right angles to one another allow a resident to maintain eye contact and re-

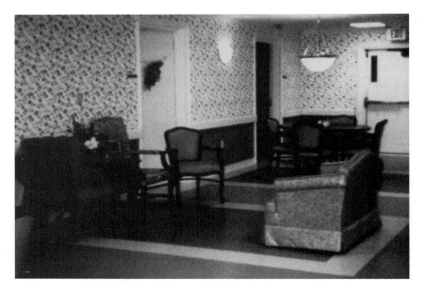

Figure 2.4.   Furniture arranged to create smaller conversational areas that promote social interaction among residents.

main in easy hearing distance. In larger spaces, it is best to group furniture in clusters to create smaller conversation areas (see Figure 2.4). Chairs placed around a table offer a natural place to engage in conversation. Books or small objects placed on the table can serve as conversation pieces.

Therapeutic Kitchens

Working in a kitchen is a familiar pattern for many residents in long-term care facilities. Residents with dementia remember many domestic activities because these activities occurred on a daily basis all of their lives. Therefore, a kitchen area that can be used by residents is an excellent backdrop for these types of activities (Figure 2.5). The things that are needed to create such an area are some kitchen cabinets, a refrigerator, a sink, and possibly a stove or hotplate (depending on what is allowed by the local fire marshal and state fire safety regulations). The area can be decorated with familiar kitchen items that might be found in your own parents' or grandparents' kitchens. These items often can be found at flea markets or garage sales. A coffee maker or bread machine can provide appropriate kitchen odors. Occasionally, residents may be able to contribute a dish to the lunch or dinner for the day. Folding napkins or sorting silverware also become natural activities in the kitchen area.

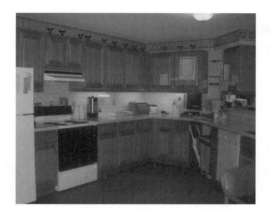

Figure 2.5. A therapeutic kitchen area enables residents to participate in familiar domestic activities.

Interactive Art as a Diversion Tactic

Researchers have argued that low-functioning residents who wander simply may be responding to various stimuli in the environment—walking toward something to which they are attracted. It is often difficult to redirect this type of wandering to make it less disruptive—these residents typically have short attention spans and do not participate in structured activities. If behavior tracking indicates that this is the case, then staff may want to make the paths used by these residents more interesting to keep them engaged and less disruptive to others. To do this, consider creating interactive art that is meant to be touched and provides a variety of sensory experiences. Tactile stimulation can be provided through different textures, parts that move, and things that can be attached or detached at a particular spot with Velcro (but are permanently attached to the artwork with string so they do not get lost) (Figure 2.6). Consider adding auditory stimulation with softly playing music boxes or greeting cards that play music when opened. Placing this art near the main wandering path may serve as an interesting diversion to wandering residents and reduce the amount of time they disturb others. The art may be hung on a wall or it could be smaller and more portable. However, if it is hung on a wall, residents may be reluctant to touch it because we are trained from an early age not to touch artwork. A visit to a local fabric or craft store may provide interesting ideas for a creative display made by staff. Also consider asking a local high school art class to create interactive art displays in your facility as a class project. "Where to Find Products" also provides some sources for interactive art.

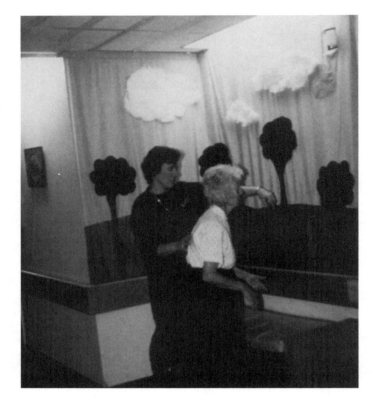

Figure 2.6.   Interactive artwork can provide a variety of sensory experiences for residents moving along a wandering path, which reduces the amount of time that they disturb others.

Orientation to Place

Finding One's Way Around

Some residents may wander because they are trying to find their way back to their rooms or to an activity. Hallways in long-term care facilities are often long and look very similar. There are several means to aid residents in finding their way around the facility. One effective way to do this is to create landmarks, or elements that provide distinctive focal points in the halls (e.g., a large quilt hung on the wall, a large clock, birds in an aviary, an aquarium). Certain walls might become landmarks themselves if they are painted a distinctive color, although this may be less effective with residents with visual impairment or those who are color-blind. If halls are to be painted different colors, the difference between colors must be strong enough to be registered by older eyes. You can test this easily by buying some yellow-tinted plastic in an art store, smearing a little petroleum jelly on one side, and looking through it at the color scheme.

In most long-term care facilities, resident bedroom doors and other doorways appear to be very similar. In addition, repetitive room layouts do not offer residents cues about which room is theirs. There are a variety of ways to help residents who appear to be wandering in search of their rooms. First, look at the resident room signage. If the signs are mounted 5 feet above the floor level, residents may not pay attention to them because they are above the residents' eye level. Lower these signs to between 40 and 48 inches above the floor. Residents who walk stooped over may benefit by having the signs mounted 10–16 inches from the floor because they may never raise their eyes to see a sign that is higher. If the signs have small lettering, then residents may not be able to read them. Sign lettering size should be at least 1 inch but preferably 2 inches high. For the best contrast, the letters should be a light color and the background a dark color. The more contrast, the more visible the sign. (See "Where to Find Products" for sources of signage that can be used for orientation.)

Another possible addition to resident room doors that may aid in orientation is a place for a photograph. Staff may have to experiment to determine which photograph each resident recognizes (e.g., him- or herself, his or her family, a favorite vacation spot, a military photo). Typed and mounted resident histories are also effective at creating distinctive room entries, as well as providing a quick way for staff to become more familiar with a new resident. Make sure that a large letter size is used so that other residents can read these histories. Shadow boxes or small curio cabinets (see Figure 2.7) that do not extend more than 4 inches into the hall are places to display items that may aid residents in finding their doors (see "Where to Find Products" for sources). Should your facility plan to purchase such cabinets, try to find ones that have nonreflective glass. Cabinets do not have to look alike; different styles also may aid a resident in finding his or her door. Using locking cabinets will prevent residents from "borrowing" items from others' cases.

Understanding the Functions of Different Spaces

Many long-term care facilities have large multipurpose rooms that are used for a variety of activities and events throughout the day (Figure 2.8). For example, a large dining room may be used for activity programming between meals. This can be disorienting to residents with dementia. Most people are

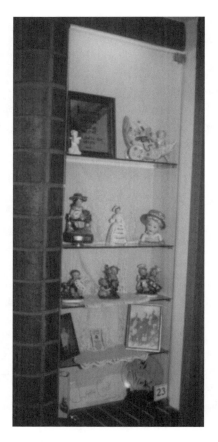

Figure 2.7. Small display cases containing personal items are used at the Corinne Dolan Alzheimer Center to help residents recognize their rooms.

accustomed to going to different places for different functions and activities. For example, religious services usually occur in a church or temple, meals occur in kitchens or dining rooms, and socializing with friends often occurs in a living room or den.

When all of these events and activities occur in the same room, residents with dementia may not understand what to do when they are in that room. The ideal solution is to have shared spaces that are used only for one purpose, for example, a dining room that is used only for meals, a craft room for art projects, and a living room for social gatherings such as discussions,

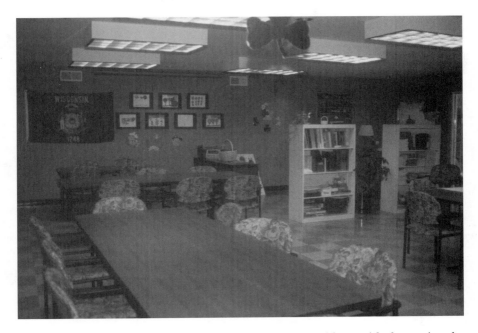

Figure 2.8.   Multipurpose rooms may be confusing to residents with dementia, who may not understand what activities are going on at various times.

sing-alongs, and videos. These single-purpose rooms should be visually distinctive in decor and furnishings so that, when a resident enters the room, he or she can determine the purpose for which the room is used.

Unfortunately, having a variety of single-purpose rooms is not possible for many facilities, but a number of things still can be done to help orient residents. For example, residents with dementia may not be able to understand verbal communications such as "it's time to eat" or "let's do some exercises." However, reinforcing verbal cues with physical cues can be effective. Examples of effective physical cues are placing tablecloths on tables to indicate that it is time for a meal. The same tape of birds chirping might be played each morning before an exercise program. For religious services, chairs can be arranged in rows rather than in a circle. Songbooks and the altar stand should appear in the room only during these services. For musical activities, consider hanging up a sign with a large musical note. This sign should be present only for these music sessions. Dinner each night might be accompanied by an olfactory cue of fresh bread being baked in a bread maker. This bread can be served with the meal each evening. Each different activity should have some type of unique, familiar cue.

Limiting Wandering into Nonresidential/Private Areas

Creating Detour Cues

Some residents who wander tend to move in straight lines, and thus often will enter rooms that are at the ends or intersections of hallways. Wandering residents often are attracted to these rooms simply because the doors are in their immediate view. This can be a problem if these rooms are someone else's bedroom or a staff/utility space that residents should not enter. If this is a problem at the facility, then staff should first determine who needs to use the door and how frequently it is used. Next, determine the cognitive abilities and interests of the residents who are wandering through the door and use this information to create a detour cue. If the door is being used inappropriately by only a few high-functioning residents, then consider hanging a sign that says, "JOHN, TURN AROUND" or "SOPHIE, DO NOT ENTER." Other possible signs to try are "STOP," "DO NOT ENTER," or "OUT OF ORDER." Other ideas about possible door treatments can be found in Chapter 3 in this volume.

Avoiding Hazardous Areas

Most facilities have storage rooms, housekeeping areas, and utility closets that residents should not enter. It is possible to reduce the interest of wandering residents in these areas. First, staff should look to see whether the signage in the buildings is the same for each room. Signs for nonresidential areas should be much smaller, and can be placed out of the direct view of residents (e.g., above the door), or in some cases, the sign can be eliminated altogether. As a general rule of thumb, rooms or areas where residents should go should have more prominent signs, and places residents should not enter should have little or no signage. Another solution is to treat the door and door frame like the surrounding wall to disguise the opening (check this with the local fire marshal first). For example, if the walls are painted, use the same paint on the door and frame to remove it from view. Adding a second doorknob that must be turned at the same time as the main knob also can discourage some residents. A gate latch on the upper portion of the door also may provide additional security. If the door is made more complicated to open, a person with dementia may lose interest in the room. These door modifications are described in further detail in Chapter 3.

Installing Wanderer Monitoring Systems

Technology also may help to track residents who wander in the facility. Some wanderer monitoring alarm/locking systems can be connected to computers. Computer software can log information about each resident who wears a tag. Originally, these systems were used to keep track of how often certain residents tried to leave the unit. However, a facility can be creative in where it places monitoring devices and can find out how often a resident enters the dining room or utility room. This information might be helpful in trying to determine which doors are the most problematic, which residents are using these doors, and when these residents are most likely to try to leave.

Excessive Walking

Residents who walk excessively may feel a need to be in motion. Providing rocking or gliding chairs may fill this need. (There are several types of these chairs on the market; manufacturers are listed in "Where to Find Products.") Be sure that the chair is stable or can be made stable while a resident is getting in or out of it. Another important feature is a construction that ensures that none of the joints and crevices in the chair will pinch a resident while it is motion.

Providing interesting things along the paths that excessive walkers use may catch their attention and cause a temporary break in their walking. One example already described in this section is interactive art. Another diversion that may work for these residents is rummaging drawers or areas. A rummaging area can be created easily by using an existing piece of furniture and stocking it with a variety of small items to sort or explore. See Chapter 4 in this volume for more ideas on creating these types of areas.

WHERE TO FIND PRODUCTS

Activity Programming

Activities Directors' Quarterly for Alzheimer's and Other Dementia Patients
470 Boston Post Road
Westen, MA 02493
(800) 800-1995

American Historic Society
Accessible through *www.SkyMall.com*
A variety of "old time" products, including bulk packages of unopened baseball cards

Briggs Corporation
Life & Enrichment Activities Catalogue
7300 Westown Parkway
West Des Moines, IA 50266
(800) 247-2343
Briggs offers a variety of activity products, including a bowling alley carpet and pins.

Eymann Publications, Inc.
Post Office Box 3577
Reno, NV 89505
(800) 354-3371
www.care4elders.com
Eymann publishes the newsletter *Activity Director's Guide*.

Geriatric Resources, Inc.
Post Office Box 239
Radium Springs, NM 88054
(800) 359-0390
www.geriatric-resources.com
The company offers *Sensory Stimulation Products*, a catalog of activity-related products, and games.

The Haworth Press
10 Alice Street
Binghamton, NY 13904-1580
(800) 342-9678
www.haworthpressinc.com
Haworth publishes *Activities, Adaptation and Aging,* a quarterly journal that provides practical research on activity programming.

Innovative Caregiving Resources
Post Office Box 17809
Salt Lake City, UT 84117-0809
(800) 249-5600
www.videorespite.com
ICR is the creator of the Video Respite videotape series that provides caregivers respite from caregiving by engaging people with dementia in age-appropriate activities.

Leisure and Aging Publications
2775 South Quincy Street, Suite 300
Arlington, VA 22206-2204
A catalog of activity-related publications is available.

NASCO
901 Janesville Avenue
Post Office Box 901
Fort Atkinson, WI 53538-0901
(800) 558-9595
www.enasco.com
Cross Creek Senior Activity Products is their catalog of activity programming products.

Potentials Development
40 Hazelwood Drive, Suite 101
Amherst, NY 14228
(800) 691-6602
A catalog of activity programming that is targeted to activity directors

United Seniors Health Cooperative
409 Third Street SW, Suite 200
Washington, DC 20024
(202) 479-6973
www.unitedseniorshealth.org
USHC offers Eldergames trivia books and picture card sets.

Radio Programming

Companion Radio
1 Fisher Road
Pittsford, NY 14534
(800) 499-4040
A satellite radio program that features age-appropriate programming

Sound Choice
14100 South Lakes Drive
Charlotte, NC 28273
(800) 788-4487
www.soundchoice.com
Reminiscing series—karaoke from 1900 to the 1940s

Interactive and Reminiscing Art

Artline
W227 North 937 Westmound Drive
Waukesha, WI 53186
(800) 795-9596
www.artline.com
Interactive and memory-based artwork

DesignXpertise Studio
1700 Mary Street
Pittsburgh, PA 15203
(412) 431-5733
www.designxpertise.com
Memory quilts and memory boxes by artist Karen Scofield

3D Interactive Art by Mardel DeBuhr Sanzotta
84 Fruitland Avenue
Painesville, OH 44077
(216) 357-7122
Tactile artwork with some interactive items

Signage

EMED Co., Inc.
Post Office Box 369
Buffalo, NY 14240-0369
(800) 442-3633
www.emedco.com
EMED offers a variety of standard facility signs and custom signage.

Graphics Systems Inc.
313 Ida
Wichita, KS 67211
(316) 267-4171
www.gsi-graphics.com

Kaltech Industries Group, Inc.
Kaltech Architectural Signage
123 West 19th Street
New York, NY 10011
(800) 435-TECH
www.kaltech.com/framset.htm
Modular sign systems that can be customized

Scott Sign Systems, Inc.
Post Office Box 1047
Tallevast, FL 34270-1047
(800) 237-9447
www.scottsigns.com

Shadow Boxes

Exposures, Inc.
Post Office Box 3615
Oshkosh, WI 54903-3615
(800) 222-4947
www.exposuresonline.com
A catalog of items for the storage and display of photographs and
mementos

Wanderer Monitoring Systems

Accutech-Wander Monitor
13555 Bishops Court, Suite 15
Brookfield, WI 53005
(414) 785-0645
A full-service, expandable system of alarms and locks

Care Trak
1031 Autumn Ridge Road
Carbondale, IL 62901
A resident wander monitor system with a tracking process

Code-Alert
3125 North 126 Street
Brookfield, WI 53005
(800) 669-9946
www.codealert.com
Code Alert is a resident wanderer monitor system that has a silent
paging option and can be connected to a computer program to log resident patterns.

EXI Wireless Inc.
13551 Commerce Parkway, Suite 100
Richmond, British Columbia V6V 2L1, Canada
(800) 667-9689
www.exi.com
EXI manufactures the RoamAlert resident wandering system.

Fidelity TeleAlarm LLC
2501 Kutztown Road
Reading, PA 19605-2961
(800) 483-0888
www.fidelitytelealarm.com
Locate 1 with optional WanderCall wireless call system

Hitec Communications
8160 Madison Avenue
Burr Ridge, IL 60521
(804) 288-6100
Integrated phone, call bell, and door monitoring system

Instantel, Inc.
808 Commerce Park Drive
Ogdensburg, NY 13669
(800) 267-9111
www.instantel.com
Instantel manufactures WatchMate, a resident wanderer monitor system with a silent paging option that can be connected to a computer program to log resident patterns.

March Networks
(formerly Elcombe Systems)
555 Legget Drive, Tower B, Suite 330
Kanata, Ontario K2K 2X3, Canada
(613) 591-8181
www.marchnetworks.com/solutions/solutions_healthcare.com
Messenger Resident Locating System with PC-based monitoring software

Senior Technologies, Inc.
Post Office Box 80238
Lincoln, NE 68501-4478
(800) 206-1044
www.seniortechnologies.com
Makes WanderGuard, a resident departure alarm system that has a silent paging option

Motion Chairs

Adden Furniture, Inc.
26 Jackson Street
Lowell, MA 01852
(508) 457-7848

Town Square Furniture, Inc.
Post Office Box 419
Hillsboro, TX 76645
(800) 356-1663
www.gliderrocker.com
Glider Rocker motion chair

Kimball Lodging Group
1180 East 16th Street
Jasper, IN 47549-1009
(800) 451-8090
www.lodging.kimball.com
Creates health care and hospitality furniture

La-Z-Boy, Inc.
1284 North Telegraph Road
Monroe, MI 48162
(734) 241-4700
www.lzbhealthcare.com
QC Collection, Wheel Care, and Recline Care lines

Sauder Manufacturing
930 West Barre Road
Archbold, OH 43502-0230
(800) 537-1530
www.saudermanufacturing.com
Offers a variety of health care-seating products

WhisperGLIDE Swing Company
10051 Kerry Court
Hugo, MN 55038
(800) 944-7737
www.whisperglide.com
WhisperGLIDE outdoor glider swing

◆ ◆ ◆

A summary sheet follows, which condenses the chapter text into a quick overview. The authors have also provided an area for you to make your own notes about your own staff and facility. Managerial staff may wish to use the summary sheets as handouts to accompany direct care staff training, or to post them by the time clock or nurses' station or include them in staff's pay envelopes.

WANDERING SUMMARY SHEET

1. Wandering is a form of walking in which a person either does not have an apparent goal (i.e., the person may not be walking to an obvious destination) or he or she is in search of someone or something that is unattainable in his or her situation.

2. People, including those with dementia, usually have reasons for their actions and behaviors. In long-term care, this is referred to as *agenda behavior.*

3. Residents may wander as a response to boredom, a roommate who is bothering them, or overstimulation from a noisy day room; because they may be trying to figure out where they are; because they may be looking for a spouse who has died or lives elsewhere; or other reasons.

4. Sometimes, residents may be able to tell staff why they are wandering (e.g., "I am looking for my daughter," or, "I am looking for my room"). Other times, staff may need to figure it out themselves (e.g., "There was so much noise in the day room that he wanted to get away"). Using the Behavior Tracking Form (see Appendix A) can help staff determine residents' reasons for leaving, and then determine how to respond.

What Staff Can Do

1. Redirect the resident with purpose. When attempting to interrupt wandering by redirection, always offer the resident a more interesting alternative. Ideally, the distraction should address his or her reason (agenda) for wandering. For example, if a resident is wandering because she is bored, find an activity that she likes to do and help her get started. If she likes to do light housekeeping, give her a broom and ask her to help sweep the hallway.

2. Schedule familiar activities. People with dementia can have a difficult time learning new things. Try to get residents who wander to participate in familiar activities that they enjoy doing.

3. Provide gender-specific activities. Although there are many activities that both men and women enjoy, some activities are more gender specific. Some men may not enjoy activities that are domestic (e.g., baking cookies). Try to provide men with activities they enjoyed throughout their life, such as woodworking, washing cars, and listening to or watching sporting events.

4. Offer snacks and drinks on a regular basis to residents who are excessive walkers. Make sure that they are wearing a comfortable pair of shoes. If you are trying to discourage their walking, make sure you offer them something to do that interests them and/or provides pleasure.

What the Environment Can Do

1. Provide cues for residents. Finding their way around may be difficult for some residents. Create signs in large lettering with their names on them. Hang pictures of them or family and friends they recognize outside their rooms.
2. Hang interactive art along the most frequently traveled routes, and place seating nearby to encourage excessive walkers to stop and rest.

YOUR NOTES

3

Attempting to Leave

People responsible for the care of residents with dementia often are required to do things that they think are in the best interests of the residents. In doing this, they may lose sight of the importance of what the resident is thinking or feeling, particularly when residents are trying to leave the unit or facility. It may be unsafe for a particular resident to leave because of his or her cognitive impairment, or the facility's policy may dictate that residents cannot leave unattended. This does not mean that residents will not want to leave the unit from time to time. This discussion of exiting or attempts to leave the unit includes occa-

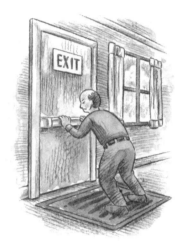

sions when residents try to leave the unit but are unsuccessful because of either locks on doors or staff intervention. The challenge is to try to determine why a resident may want or try to leave, and how staff can keep them from wanting to leave, enable them to leave the unit in a safe manner, or offer them something of interest to do instead of leaving.

WHY RESIDENTS MIGHT WANT TO LEAVE

There are as many reasons why residents of long-term care facilities may want to leave the unit or facility in which they live as there are reasons why we do not want to stay in the same building day in and day out. Their reasons may be as simple as looking out the window near an exit door and seeing that it is a beautiful day, and wanting to feel the sun on their skin and the breeze in the air. Another possibility is that they are bored with their current environment and want to go somewhere else. At other times, residents may have a more specific reason for wanting to leave. For example, they may want to return home to live, or, depending on their orientation to time and place, they may think that they need to go to work. If our friends gave any of these reasons for wanting to leave, we would not think to question them. All of these reasons make perfect sense. Yet, so often we just redirect residents away from the door without addressing their reason(s) for wanting to leave.

Whereas many residents have reasons for trying to leave, there are others whose attempts to leave are unintentional. This may take the form of *shadowing* or simply exploring. Shadowing occurs when a resident's actions are triggered by the actions of another person. For example, the resident simply follows another person who is leaving the unit. Residents who are simply exploring may not be attempting to leave at all, but may be attracted to a shiny silver door handle or elevator button and press it (possibly setting off an alarm) just out of curiosity (Dickinson, McLain-Kark, & Marshall-Baker, 1995).

PATTERNS OF LEAVING

Before you can determine the best intervention for each resident, you must determine what triggers their attempts to leave and if there are any patterns to the behavior. One of the most effective ways to gather this information is to implement a behavior tracking process similar to that described in Chapter 1 of this volume. A Behavior Tracking Form has been provided in Appendix A that you may use as is or revise to suit your needs.

The person who conducts the tracking process should explain to staff members the value of talking to residents about why they want to leave. This information is valuable to record on the tracking form so that interventions can be directed at addressing the residents' underlying desires. Furthermore, by talking with residents, staff are validating their feelings and helping them to know that their feelings are important. This personal attention may be enough to deter a resident from trying to leave again. It also can be useful to talk to family members to find out if the resident had a history of leaving (e.g., wandering away from home after the onset of dementia) or to explore any previous daily routines that could trigger his or her leaving (e.g., always took a walk in the morning, left for work at the same time). Relatives also may be able to suggest other strategies to deter their family member from trying to exit. It is also important to talk to the direct care staff from each shift about any strategies that they have found effective.

DETERMINING APPROPRIATE INTERVENTIONS

A number of interventions can be implemented in response to unwanted exiting of residents. Ideally, the facility should provide a means for residents to be able to leave, either into a secured courtyard or to another part of the facility. Everyone, regardless of cognitive status, still wants the freedom to make choices. Unfortunately, in long-term care settings residents often lose many of their freedoms; therefore, it is important that facilities make an effort to give residents as much freedom as possible.

A useful approach to exiting is the agenda behavior approach (Rader, Doan, & Schwab, 1985), which suggests that people do things for a reason. Thus, it is important to determine why the resident is doing something before trying to change that behavior (Figure 3.1). A more detailed description of this process is provided in Chapter 1 of this volume. Ideas for specific interventions related to decreasing and responding to attempts to leave the unit are offered in "What Staff Can Do" and "What the Environment Can Do."

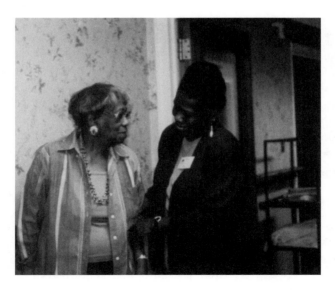

Figure 3.1.   It is important to determine a resident's reasons for attempting to leave the facility before trying to intervene.

WHAT STAFF CAN DO

Addressing Patterns of Exiting

It is important to know whether there are patterns to residents' exiting. You may already be familiar with your residents' reasons. If you are not, then it will be helpful to implement a tracking process for exiting behaviors. Once this is done, it is important to look at the information gathered and determine how it can affect the programming on the unit. Look at the tracking forms for patterns in exiting. If a number of residents tend to exit at a similar time each day, then staff should try to engage these residents in an activity at this time. When a resident has a tendency to want to leave at the same time each day, try to involve him or her in a one-to-one activity or conversation at this time. It is also important to look at the underlying needs that may be influencing residents to want to leave. Staff should try to incorporate these reasons into social programming and activities. A few common reasons for leaving and suggestions for interventions are listed in Table 3.1.

Understandably, group activities cannot please everybody all of the time. Yet, there may be small groups of residents who enjoy the same interests or have similar backgrounds (e.g., teachers, homemakers, golfers). Furthermore, the residents who leave the unit are likely to be some of the same ones who wander. Because wanderers tend to be less social, these residents can particularly benefit from one-to-one interactions with staff. Conversing with a resident should be considered an important part of the program because social conversation is a normal part of everyday life for most people. Therefore, the goals of such interactions are to add meaning and quality to the lives of the residents.

Methods for Decreasing Exiting

Redirecting

Redirecting a resident who is attempting to leave can be effective in some cases and will be most successful when the redirection is aimed at the interests of the specific resident. For instance, initiating a simple task or activity that the resident enjoys is more likely to be successful than just directing the resident back to his or her room or to the day room (Figure 3.2). For known exiters, find a task or activity that each seems to enjoy or feels useful in doing, and make sure that all staff know about this intervention. If possible, this task/activity should address the resident's underlying reason for wanting to

Table 3.1. Reasons for residents' attempts to leave and suggested
interventions

Reason for attempting to leave	Related activities for intervention
To go to work	If some residents worked in an office, create an officelike space where residents can do office tasks (e.g., sorting mail, stuffing envelopes, filing); if they worked in other settings, then try to re-create some of them and organize related tasks for each.
To get home to children	Plan cooking and baking activities, which are home-related activities; arrange intergenerational programs with preschool or elementary school students to give residents exposure to children.
To be outside	Plan walks, picnics, and other activities to be held outside during good weather; keep in mind that some residents enjoy the ability to go outside regardless of the weather.

leave. It is helpful to keep the necessary props close to the exit that the resident most frequently uses. Tasks or activities that may work for some residents
include

- Flipping through photo albums supplied by the resident's family
- Folding towels, napkins, or tablecloths
- Listening to favorite music
- Going through baseball cards
- Working on jigsaw puzzles (keep eyesight, finger dexterity, and cogni-
  tive level of the resident in mind when selecting number and size of
  pieces; also, try to find puzzles that are adult in nature)
- Cutting coupons

These are only some general ideas, and staff who work closest with a particular resident may be able to suggest something that is unique to that resident.
(Also see "Where to Find Products" for sources of activity programming.)

Avoiding Residents' Seeing Others Leave

Sometimes residents' desire to leave may stem from seeing other people leave
or hearing others talking about leaving. This is a factor that staff have some
ability to control. Emphasize the importance of leaving the unit as unobtrusively as possible to staff as well as visitors. You may want to make an effort to
distract some residents from the exit around the time of shift changes to re-

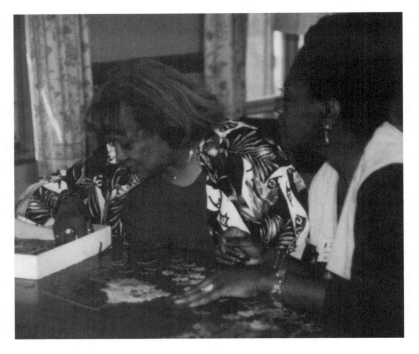

Figure 3.2.   Engaging a resident in an activity he or she enjoys helps to redirect that resident's attempts to leave the facility.

duce the chances of them trying to leave. Also, ask staff to limit discussions among themselves about leaving and going home when residents are around. Staff should try to keep their coats in a location close to the exit or off the unit, so that residents will not see them putting on their coats to leave.

When a Resident Successfully Leaves a Unit

Despite best efforts, there may be occasions when a resident is successful in leaving the unit or facility. When this happens, it is important to have a plan of action in place. This plan of action should include a step-by-step process that staff initiate to find the resident. The process should begin with a thorough, systematic search of the unit on which the resident lives because residents sometimes find inconspicuous hiding places on the unit.

The plan of action for finding a missing resident should be known by all staff of the facility because the resident may have left the unit and gone into another part of the building. You also may want to alert surrounding businesses and residences as to whom to contact if they suspect that they see a resident of the facility. It is particularly useful to have wandering/exiting residents wear identification bracelets that neighboring people could recognize. For more ideas, contact your local Alzheimer's Association to learn about their Safe Return program and to borrow videos related to unsafe wandering (see "Where to Find Products" at the end of this chapter).

WHAT THE ENVIRONMENT CAN DO

Minimizing Confinement and Regulating Stimulation

Many residents try to leave the unit because they feel a sense of confinement. This is understandable because most people do not like to feel locked in. The ability of many residents to go to different places is reduced when they move into a shared living setting, particularly if they move onto a secured unit. People who are used to being independent and running their own lives may resent being told that they can no longer do certain things or go various places. They may perceive themselves as still being capable of living independently and may not realize that restrictions are in place for their own safety. The ideal solution is to create a setting in which the residents can come and go from the unit into safe and secure indoor and outdoor spaces. This does not mean that every exit needs to be open and accessible because there are usually hazards in or near every facility. When the unit is partially secured, an adjacent courtyard is the best solution. The knowledge that they can leave when they wish may address some residents' agenda behavior.

Having an outdoor space that residents can go to freely supports their sense of independence. Care should be taken when developing outdoor

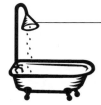

Leaving the Unit

Research at one facility demonstrated a variety of negative consequences when the exit doors to the courtyard were secured. Wandering, walking with intent (or pacing), and agitation were significantly more common when the exit doors were locked. When the doors were unlocked, a number of residents pushed the door to see if it would open, or held the door with one hand, stepped outside, looked around, and then quietly came back inside. The goal, apparently, was not to go out but to know that they were not confined (Namazi & Johnson, 1992).

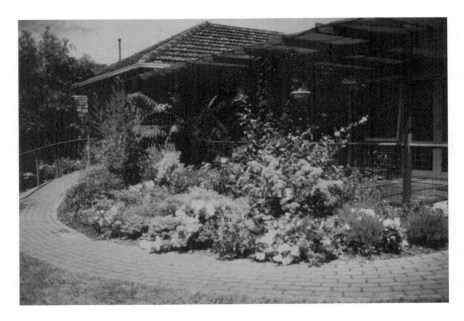

Figure 3.3.   Creating an outdoor space that is both secure and interesting provides residents who attempt to leave with a place to go outside the facility.

spaces to ensure that they are both secure and interesting (Figure 3.3). If the area is not surrounded by buildings, then fences should be at least 7 feet but preferably 8 feet high. When selecting a fence, make sure that it is difficult to climb. If the view on the other side of the fence is interesting, then a solid fence may minimize residents' desire to leave. Table 3.2 compares different types of fencing. Plants should be nontoxic, and some should be planted in raised beds to allow nonambulatory residents a chance to garden (see Volume 4, Appendix C for a list of nontoxic plants). Walking paths should be as level as possible and provide places where residents can sit and rest. In warm climates, shade from trees or shelters makes outdoor environments usable year-round. Courtyards that provide shelter from winds and some direct sunlight are preferred in northern climates. Do not assume that residents will not want to go outside in the middle of winter. Residents who have lived all of their lives in northern climates are accustomed to dealing with winter weather.

If creating such an area adjacent to the unit is impossible, then try to schedule regular visits or activities outdoors. Another idea is to invite residents to visit or attend activities in other areas of the facility. These are wonderful

Table 3.2. Comparison of fencing options

	Stockade	Chain link	Aluminum picket	Masonry wall
Description	Stockade fences are usually wood slats that completely obscure the view beyond.	Woven wire stretched on metal posts; can be covered in green or black PVC or painted	Metal posts and rails that resemble wrought iron fencing	Stone, concrete block, or brick wall
Pros	Hides view that might be attractive to residents with dementia Wood fencing has a warm and residential appearance. Gates can easily appear to blend into fence	Can have a less heavy look and can look less confining than stockade fencing Vegetation can hide or obscure this fence over time. With PVC coating, this fence can visually recede and allows views beyond Fairly inexpensive	Elegant, lacy appearance Can select a design that avoids handholds and footholds for climbing and hides gates Virtually no maintenance	Difficult to climb Most are maintenance free Hides any desirable view that would be attractive to residents with dementia
Cons	Can appear heavy and confining for small spaces Depending on the spacing of the boards, can be easily climbable Depending on the length, can be moderately expensive and requires periodic maintenance	Tall chain fencing can have an institutional feel Without PVC coating, can be a source of glare Can be climbed because of the abundance of hand- and footholds Gates stand out visually Will not obscure views	Will not obscure views Expensive Improper design and selection can make this fence easy to climb and can make gates noticeable	Can be expensive Gates stand out visually Heavy and can obscure light
Suggestions for use	To obscure a desirable view or dangerous area When a moderate cost, solid fence is needed	When cost is a primary consideration When a pleasant view beyond is desirable to be seen	When appearance is a primary concern When a view does not need to be obscured	When a view needs to be obscured In a relatively open space that has plenty of sun and air

47

opportunities for volunteer and family member participation. Just being able to leave the unit may alleviate some residents' sense of confinement.

Residents may be trying to leave the unit because they are looking for something interesting to do. If it is known, or tracking sheets indicate, that residents attempt to leave the unit when there is little going on, staff need to develop a more diverse activity program that keeps more residents engaged for longer periods of time over the course of the day. This does not mean there has to be a staffed activity going on at all times (although many units do not have nearly enough structured activities). Ensure that there are both opportunities and props to encourage people to engage in a variety of individual or small group activities—activities that do not necessarily require ongoing staff direction. Many residents will find it hard to initiate these activities on their own, but they may be able to continue with an activity once it is set up and started for them. For instance, an aide walking by the residents may easily be able to encourage them to start a project of folding towels or get a group singing without supervising the entire activity. (See Chapter 4 in this volume for other ideas for creating sensory stimulation areas.)

Recognizing that many people with dementia are easily overwhelmed, it is also important to pay attention to how much stimulation occurs on the unit. It is possible that a resident is trying to leave the unit to find a quiet place. If this appears to be an issue, then it is probably worth doing a separate assessment of the stimulation level on the unit. The Sensory Stimulation Assessment form in Appendix B of this volume can be used to conduct such an assessment. Over the course of several days, staff can use this form to record exactly what is occurring on the unit every hour. The person doing the assessment should close his or her eyes and listen for 30–60 seconds, then write down every sound he or she heard (including people, machines, and public address systems), as well as the loudness of the sounds. Then the assessor should look around and record how many people are visible, how many are walking, and how many are engaged in other movements or activities. Also, he or she should record the number of carts or other objects in the hallways.

Once you have a record of the standard sources of stimulation, determine which ones are most common, most annoying, or both and then develop a plan to minimize or eliminate these sources. Some examples might include determining whether the public address system is absolutely necessary on this unit. In some facilities, overhead announcements are limited to emergencies only. Train staff to respond to and turn off call bells immediately, rather than letting them sound for long periods of time. Of course, the facility must have adequate staffing so that staff are able to respond quickly. Some

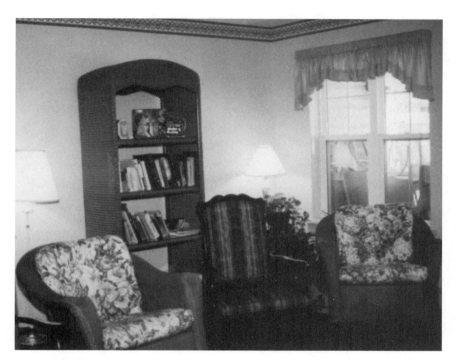

Figure 3.4.   Create a quiet space for calming overstimulated residents who would otherwise attempt to leave the unit.

alarm sounds (not fire and emergency alarms, but other door alarms) can be changed to chimes rather than an obnoxious buzzer. Staff should be able to adjust to responding to a chime instead of an obnoxious alarm and will likely welcome the change. Encourage staff to avoid yelling to each other across the unit or room. Must laundry and housekeeping carts be used on the unit during shift change? Can some of these activities be done at other times of the day, such as during the night shift? Alternatively, determine whether some of these everyday events, such as helping to distribute the laundry, can become activities for understimulated residents.

If it is difficult to lower excessive stimulation on the unit, then staff should consider placing overstimulated residents in a quieter place where they can spend some time during, or just before, the periods when they try to leave the unit (Figure 3.4). An enclosed lounge, if available, can be used as a quiet area on the unit. This room should not have a public address system speaker, and television and radio use should be adjusted to the needs of the individual residents. Music might be made available by residents' using headphones.

Sheers or translucent shades can be used to soften light from windows. Provide soft, subdued lighting from table or floor lamps instead of overhead lights, and use comfortable furniture and several throw pillows to decorate the room. Pleasant background noise may come from a small indoor tabletop waterfall or aquarium. This room can be used as a quiet area to calm an agitated resident or as a respite area for those who are overstimulated. Residents may learn to seek out this area when they are feeling overwhelmed.

Modifying Doorways to Reduce Exiting

Making Doors Look Less Like Doors

Another strategy to minimize residents' leaving is to make the exit doors look less obviously like doors. The facility must check with the local fire marshal about regulations pertaining to disguising doors before making any changes. Some facilities have painted a mural across the door so that it is not readily seen as a door. If the door is flanked by windows, then try continuing the window treatment (such as cafe curtains) from adjacent windows across the door. A less extreme example (which might meet more fire codes) is to decorate the exit door exactly like the surrounding wall. If the wall is painted blue, then paint the door and the frame the same color. If there is wainscoting or other treatment on the bottom of the wall, and paint or wallpaper above, then continue it across the door (Figure 3.5). Paint the door handle or panic bar to match the door's color, if possible. This strategy works best on doors that are not used frequently by anyone. Handrails typically stop at doorways, so having them continue across the doors can decrease the likelihood of residents' perceiving them as exits. Remember that this must not impede the use of the door in an emergency.

Reducing View to Other Side of Door

Another common reason that residents try to leave the unit is that what they see on the other side of the door interests them. When tracking residents who are trying to leave the unit, note whether there are windows in or adjacent to the doors that may provide views to interesting areas such as outside spaces, parking lots, streets with cars, or people on other units. When possible within the parameters of local and regional fire codes, minimize visibility through these doors to the other side, particularly if the view is likely to be of interest to residents. Check with the local fire marshal to determine whether windows are required in the doors, and, if they are, whether they can be covered with curtains on at least one side. Decreasing residents' visual access to potentially

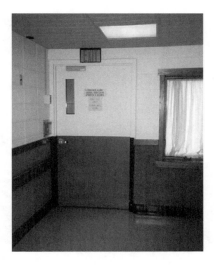

Figure 3.5. Wainscoting or other wall treatments should be continued across the exit to disguise it.

interesting but inappropriate areas may decrease their desire to leave via these doors. Also, consider dimming the lighting around these exits. Many residents with dementia are less likely to approach a spot that is darker than the surrounding area.

Other Door Modifications

Another strategy to consider is placing a strip of fabric, approximately 12–15 inches high, across the door at the height of the door handle (Figure 3.6). Velcro strips are stitched to the ends of the fabric and tacked onto the wall adjacent to the door frame. In states that require less than 5 pounds of pressure to open an exit door, this treatment may be approved by the local fire marshal, particularly when instructions on how to remove the fabric and open the door in an emergency are placed nearby. These instructions should be written so it looks as though there are several steps that must be taken to open the door. This modification will be most successful on doors that are not used often, because if residents see staff undoing the fabric to go through the doorway, they may soon start to do the same.

There may also be ways of removing redundant signs from exit doors. Check with the local fire marshal to determine whether one of the signs can be removed if the exit door is labeled in more than one way. If signs cannot

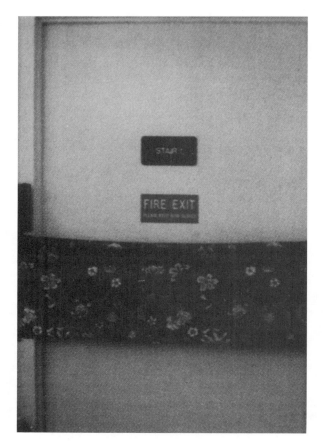

Figure 3.6.   A strip of fabric placed across a door at the
height of the handle may deter residents from trying to
exit through that door.

be removed, then find out whether they can be placed higher on the door
and out of residents' direct view. Other entry deterrents include placing a vel-
vet rope, similar to those used in movie theaters, in front of a door that residents should not use. Placing a dark mat on the floor in front of the door may
keep some residents from approaching the door because the dark mat can
look like a hole (Figure 3.7).

All of these interventions should be reviewed by the local fire marshal
before they are implemented. It is important to experiment to determine
what works best for your situation. When something does not work the first
time or stops being effective, try it again later.

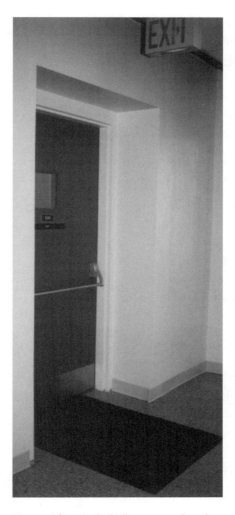

Figure 3.7. A dark floor mat placed at the bottom of a door may keep some residents away from the door because the mat looks to them like a hole in the floor.

Cognitive Locks

Knowing that people with dementia find it more difficult to process and make sense of new situations, it is possible to make opening doors more difficult without including actual locks. Adding a second doorknob that must be turned at the same time as the main knob to open the door can discourage some residents. A gate latch on the upper portion of the door also may provide additional security. A resident with dementia may give up on trying to use a door that is complicated to open. Many of these types of locks will not be allowed on doors that serve as fire exits, but they certainly can be used on doors to utility rooms or other areas you want to discourage residents from entering. They do, however, also make the doors harder for staff to open when their hands are full.

Signage

Numerous facilities have used different signs to discourage residents from using exits inappropriately. The most common sign is probably a STOP sign, although this may not be effective. As one resident said, when asked what the sign meant, "First you stop, then you go through." Other signs to consider include DO NOT ENTER, OUT OF ORDER, and USE OTHER DOOR. Other facilities have worked to understand why a particular resident attempted to leave and developed a sign to address that resident. For example, one facility posted a sign that read TRAINS NOT RUNNING to deter one resident. Another hung a sign that read MARY, TURN AROUND. When developing signs and evaluating their effectiveness, create them on paper first using simple language or graphics. When you find a sign that works, consider having it professionally made so that its appearance is more appealing and less makeshift. You may be able to find the sign available commercially (see "Where to Find Products" for sources).

Security Systems

Lock and Alarm Systems

Many facilities place some type of alarm or locking system on their exit doors. Door security systems have three basic components—alarms, locking systems, and activation systems—each of which can be configured in several ways. Before any decisions regarding door security systems are made, check with the local fire marshal, licensing agency, or both to determine what is allowed.

By itself, an alarm only alerts staff that someone is attempting to leave the unit, and usually requires staff to go to the exit to retrieve the resident. Some systems allow the alarm to be disengaged at the nurses' station (meaning staff need not physically go to the exit door), whereas others can be disengaged only at the exit door. Alarms can be configured in various ways to sound or not sound (see "System Alterations" later in this section). If the facility is using or thinking about installing an alarm system, then staff should consider carefully whether the alarms need to be sirenlike, as they typically are. Alternatives that are less disruptive to other residents and ongoing activities include staff beepers, which are quiet or silent, or alarms configured to sound a chime or play a short tune.

The types of locking systems that are allowed in different states and for different levels of care vary depending on various codes and regulations. In many states, electromagnetic locks are allowed provided that they are tied into the fire alarm system and automatically release in an emergency. Other states allow electromagnetic locks only if they are configured to release if the panic bar is depressed for 15–30 seconds. Typically, an alarm sounds when the bar is depressed, which alerts staff to a potential unauthorized exit. The latter system has several disadvantages. First, the alarm is usually intrusive and disruptive to other residents and ongoing activities. Second, because the door will open after 15–30 seconds, a staff member must stop what he or she is doing and go to the door and retrieve the resident. Chronic exit seekers can disrupt many activities.

Both alarms and locks can be activated or deactivated in several different ways. The most basic system is nonadjustable (it always sounds when the door is opened or is always locked except in an emergency), so there is no way to de-activate the alarm/lock. The next level is a system in which the alarm/lock can be disengaged temporarily at the door by either a push-button keypad or one or two simple buttons that are usually somewhat hidden or disguised, or by using a key. If a keypad sys-tem is selected, then be sure that the combina-tion can be reset by the facility, and that the sys-tem does not require someone from the manu-facturer to set a new com-bination. A third system is operated with a remote (i.e., not at the door) activation/de-activation switch. This switch al-lows the doors to be unlocked/not alarmed at certain times but not at oth-ers. A remote switch system often is used on doors to courtyards so that the door can be unlocked during the day but locked/alarmed at night or in bad weather.

Wanderer Monitoring Systems

Various systems to monitor wandering residents are based on tags that residents wear (see "Where to Find Products"). These fall into two categories. The first usually is set up to sound the alarm or lock the door when a resident wearing a tag approaches a monitored door. There are both practical and ethical challenges to this type of system:

- When a resident wearing a tag approaches a door and activates the locking alarm system, someone who is authorized to leave (or enter) the unit cannot unlock the door.
- A tag on a resident who happens to be in the area of a monitored door may set off the alarm when someone opens the door. This unnecessary alarm may disturb the entire unit, particularly if it occurs regularly.
- Tagging a resident violates the dignity of the resident, especially when tags are large and obtrusive.

Despite these limitations, tag systems can provide the greatest amount of freedom to most of the residents and therefore should be considered in some situations.

The second type of tag system is specifically designed to track a resident who has left the facility. This system may or may not signal that the resident has left and helps find the resident who has left. Some residents are creative about finding ways to leave a unit despite precautions. It is important to be able to locate the resident outside the facility. All facilities should have in place a protocol for searching for lost residents. If the facility does not have such a protocol in place, then refer to "What Staff Can Do" for more information on how to set up one. In addition, if one or more residents manage to get out of the building repeatedly, consider investing in a tracking system. Residents who are known to be at risk for leaving the facility wear a wire-based tag, which is usually hidden in a belt or watch. This tag acts like a homing device and can be tracked via radio frequency for up to a mile away, identifying which direction the resident has gone. These systems work best in wide, open areas. Urban areas with many buildings can cause the system to function poorly.

System Alterations

Your facility may already have in place some type of wanderer monitoring or security system. However, technology has improved many of these systems so that they offer many additional benefits. Wanderer monitors now have much less obtrusive tags (devices that trigger alarms or locks) that are not as degrading to residents. Some tags look almost like watches or jewelry or can be hidden in the seams of clothes or in belts. Other systems can be altered so that they do not set off a loud alarm that disturbs other residents. A chime can be set to sound only at the nurses' station, or a signal can be sent to a pager that is worn by staff. This type of system is ideal because it provides a great deal of information without cluttering the environment with sounds. Even without major reconfigurations, some of the loud buzzers or sirens on alarms can be replaced with a chime or a musical tune. Some systems display a door code in a conspicuous place that allows staff to know which door has been used. Facilities that have a system with loud alarms can contact the manufacturer's representative to discuss ways of modifying the system to be less obtrusive. Some systems can be connected to a computer to keep track of all incidents related to exiting.

Elevators as Specific Problem Areas

Elevators on long-term care units can be exits for residents who are attempting to leave the facility. Staff must review this problem by determining whether residents are specifically calling for the elevator and leaving or just walking on the elevator when the doors open, and then look for an appropriate intervention. The problem is harder to address when residents are walking into the elevator car when the doors open. One inexpensive solution is to place a black mat in front of the elevator, which may deter some residents from entering. If this does not work, then consider using a wanderer monitor system. Some alarm and locking systems have components that disable, lock, or alarm elevator doors.

Several strategies can make elevator call buttons less visible or obvious. One is to hang a sign or piece of fabric over the button. Staff and visitors can learn where to push without having to lift the fabric. One facility adapted a small curio box by removing the bottom of the box and placing it on the wall so that it covered the call buttons. To call the elevator, staff first checked to make sure no residents were in the hall watching, then reached under the box and pushed the button. Another facility created a metal plate with small holes in it and placed it over the call buttons. Pressing the button required inserting a pen or pencil through the hole.

Elevator doors also can be disguised using paint or wallpaper to make them blend in with the walls on either side. More sophisticated resident tagging systems can keep elevator doors from opening when chronic exit seekers are adjacent to the elevator. If residents have access to elevators but you do not want them to go to some floors, such as the basement, then consider covering that button in the elevator. For example, metal buttons easily could be covered with a magnet. Employing this strategy requires that the covering be removed before the button can be pushed.

Windows as Specific Problem Areas

Some residents have been known to open windows and climb out in an attempt to leave the unit. It is difficult to know to what extent they realize what they are doing. Of course, staff should find out why these residents are leaving and address their underlying needs. However, there are also ways to make the windows both secure and operable, allowing residents to choose to get some fresh air in their rooms. Hardware stores sell simple window locks (usually marketed for security from burglars) that limit how far a window can be opened. Some of these have a small knob the position of which can be changed to allow the window to be opened all the way, while others require a key; the latter are probably safer. Check with the local fire marshal and licensing agency for any restriction codes.

WHERE TO FIND PRODUCTS

Identification Bracelets and Videos

Alzheimer's Association (national headquarters)
919 North Michigan Avenue, Suite 1100
Chicago, IL 60611-1676
(800) 272-3900
www.alz.org
Safe Return program, which provides identification products, including bracelets

Activity Programming

American Historic Society
Accessible through *www.SkyMall.com*
A variety of "old time" products, includes bulk packages of unopened baseball cards

Briggs Corporation
Life & Enrichment Activities Catalog
7300 Westown Parkway
West Des Moines, IA 50266
(800) 247-2343
A variety of activity products, including a bowling alley carpet and pins

Eymann Publications, Inc.
Post Office Box 3577
Reno, NV 89505
(800) 354-3371
www.care4elders.com
Publisher of the newsletter *Activity Director's Guide*

Geriatric Resources, Inc.
11636 North Dona Ana Road
Las Cruces, NM 88005
(800) 359-0390
www.geriatric-resources.com
The company offers *Sensory Stimulation Products,* a catalog of activity-related products, and games.

The Haworth Press
10 Alice Street
Binghamton, NY 13904-1580
(800) 342-9678
www.haworthpressinc.com
Publisher of *Activities, Adaptation and Aging,* a quarterly journal that provides practical research on activity programming

Innovative Caregiving Resources
Post Office Box 17809
Salt Lake City, UT 84117-0809
(801) 249-5600
www.videorespite.com
ICR is the creator of the Video Respite videotape series, which provides caregivers respite from caregiving by engaging people with dementia in age-appropriate activities.

Leisure and Aging Publications
2775 South Quincy Street, Suite 300
Arlington, VA 22206-2204
A catalog of activity-related publications is available.

NASCO
901 Janesville Avenue
Post Office Box 901
Fort Atkinson, WI 53538-0901
(800) 558-9595
www.enasco.com
Cross Creek Senior Activity Products is their catalog of activity programming products.

Potentials Development
40 Hazelwood Drive, Suite 101
Amherst, NY 14228
(800) 691-6602
A catalog of activity programming that is targeted to activity directors

United Seniors Health Cooperative
409 Third Street SW, Suite 200
Washington, DC 20024
(202) 479-6973
www.unitedseniorshealth.org
USHC offers Eldergames trivia books and picture card sets.

Radio Programming

Companion Radio
1 Fisher Road
Pittsford, NY 14534
(800) 499-4040
A satellite radio program featuring age-appropriate programming

Sound Choice
14100 South Lakes Drive
Charlotte, NC 28273
(800) 788-4487
www.soundchoice.com
Reminiscing series—karaoke from 1900 to the 1940s

Signage

EMED Co., Inc.
Post Office Box 369
Buffalo, NY 14240-0369
(800) 442-3633
www.emedco.com
EMED offers a variety of standard facility signs and custom signage.

Graphics Systems Inc.
313 Ida
Wichita, KS 67211
(316) 267-4171
www.gsi-graphics.com

Kaltech Architectural Signage
123 West 19th Street
New York, NY 10011
(800) 435-TECH
www.kaltech.com/framset.htm
Modular sign systems that can be customized

Scott Sign Systems, Inc.
Post Office Box 1047
Tallevast, FL 34270-1047
(800) 237-9447
www.scottsigns.com

Wanderer Monitoring Systems

Accutech-Wander Monitor
13555 Bishops Court, Suite 15
Brookfield, WI 53005
(414) 785-0645
A full-service, expandable system of alarms and locks

Care Trak
1031 Autumn Ridge Road
Carbondale, IL 62901
A resident wander monitor system with a tracking process

Code Alert
3125 North 126 Street
Brookfield, WI 53005
(800) 669-9946
www.codealert.com
Code Alert is a resident wanderer monitor system that has a silent paging option and can be connected to a computer program to log resident patterns.

EXI Wireless, Inc.
13551 Commerce Parkway, Suite 100
Richmond, British Columbia V6V 2L1, Canada
(800) 667-9689
www.exi.com
EXI manufactures the RoamAlert resident wandering system.

Fidelity TeleAlarm LLC
2501 Kutztown Road
Reading, PA 19605-2961
(800) 483-0888
www.fidelitytelealarm.com
Locate 1 with optional WanderCall wireless call system

Hitec Communications
8160 Madison Avenue
Burr Ridge, IL 60521
(804) 288-6100
Integrated phone, call bell, and door monitoring system

Instantel, Inc
808 Commerce Park Drive
Ogdensburg, NY 13669
(800) 267-9111
www.instantel.com
Instantel manufactures WatchMate, a resident wanderer monitor system that has a silent paging option and can be connected to a computer program to log resident patterns.

March Networks
(formerly Elcombe Systems)
555 Legget Drive, Tower B, Suite 330
Post Office Box 72088
Kanata, Ontario K2K 2X3, Canada
(613) 591-8181, (800) 563-5564
www.marchnetworks.com/solutions/solutions_healthcare.com
Messenger Resident Locating System with PC-based monitoring software

Senior Technologies, Inc.
Post Office Box 80238
Lincoln, NE 68501-4478
(800) 206-1044
www.seniortechnologies.com
Makes WanderGuard, a resident departure alarm system that has a silent paging option

◆ ◆ ◆

A summary sheet follows, which condenses the chapter text into a quick overview. The authors have also provided an area for you to make your own notes about your own staff and facility. Managerial staff may wish to use the summary sheets as handouts to accompany direct care staff training, or to post them by the time clock or nurses' station or include them in staff's pay envelopes.

ATTEMPTING TO LEAVE SUMMARY SHEET

What Staff Can Do

1. Make time to talk to the residents and get to know them (e.g., go with a resident for a short walk outside when she notices that it is a nice day and talk with her about her life). This knowledge adds meaning and quality to the residents' lives and your work. It will also make it easier for you to find effective ways to distract them from leaving.

2. Redirect residents from leaving. Always offer a resident something to do that relates to his or her agenda behavior. For example, a resident who wants to go home to cook dinner may enjoy cooking activities or setting tables at the facility; a resident who wants to see his family members may enjoy looking through his photo album.

3. Engage residents whenever possible. Residents who participate in events and activities tend to wander less. It is everyone's responsibility, not just the activities staff's, to make sure that residents enjoy a meaningful and high quality of life. If your schedule does not allow for one-to-one activities, see what you can do with the time you have. Try these suggestions:
    *   Start a group singing as you pass by.
    *   Begin a towel-folding project while you are distributing laundry.
    *   Seat two residents together who enjoy socializing at a table with coffee.
    *   Brush a resident's hair or assist with a manicure.
    *   Help a resident stay in touch with relatives by writing letters dictated by them.
    *   Accompany a resident to the gift or sundries shop.

4. Be unobtrusive when leaving a secured unit. Avoid talking about leaving or plans to leave. If possible, do not put your coat on in direct view of residents.

5. Know your facility's procedure for locating a resident who has left the facility or unit inappropriately.

What the Environment Can Do

1. Try to create a secure outdoor area where residents can come and go as they please, even if it is only a small area.

2. Accompany residents to areas off the unit and outside when possible.

3. Give residents a vacation from overstimulation, especially those with dementia because they are easily distracted by noise and commotion:
    *   Turn off alarms and call bells as soon as possible.
    *   Avoid yelling across a room.
    *   Turn down loud radios and televisions.
    *   Learn to recognize when a resident is stressed and assist him or her in moving to a quiet area.

YOUR NOTES

4

Rummaging and Hoarding

Rummaging, or going through other residents' belongings, is a common complaint in long-term care facilities. Residents who are cognitively intact often are offended by this behavior and become frustrated when the resident with dementia will not listen to their requests to leave them and their belongings alone. Staff also may become frustrated when the nurses' station becomes the target of rummagers. It is easy to feel that nothing can be put down and left for a moment without it disappearing. There are also legitimate health and safety concerns when residents hoard perishable food or condiments such as salt and sugar.

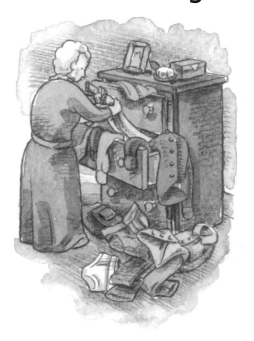

Keeping track of all of these items can take a great deal of staff time—time that might be more productively used doing other activities. Rummaging and hoarding are also difficult behaviors to control because there are so many places where residents can rummage and so many items that can be hoarded.

For many facilities, the solution to dealing with rummaging has been to try to limit the spaces to which the residents have access. Closets and dressers are locked, storage areas are secured, and shared spaces such as activity rooms and lounges have little in the way of things to rummage through. Unfortunately, this type of approach is unlikely to curb residents' desire to rummage and only encourages them to become more creative in finding places to rummage.

As with all other disruptive behaviors, the first step is to determine why residents are rummaging or hoarding. Staff who are uncertain of these reasons can keep a log tracking who, what (both what are they rummaging through or hoarding, and what else is happening on the unit), when, where, and why. Use the Behavior Tracking Form in Appendix A of this volume or make your own. The goal is to determine what prompts residents to engage in this behavior. As with the other behaviors described in this volume, different factors may motivate rummaging and hoarding; some common reasons are discussed here. Success in developing effective interventions is a direct result of being able to identify the underlying agenda of the resident and address that need. Simply removing opportunities for rummaging is unlikely to be successful.

It is also important to think about whether the rummaging is really a problem. If it keeps a person happily engaged for 30 minutes or an hour, then is it really so terrible that their drawers are disorganized? Of course, if a resident is determined to rummage in someone else's room, then the behavior is a problem.

COMMON REASONS FOR RUMMAGING

The majority of long-term care settings are fairly sterile and lack sources of tactile stimulation. In comparison, a typical home, such as those that residents came from, likely were filled—some might say overstuffed—with objects. Rugs on the floor, throw pillows, small blankets over the backs of the sofas, lace doilies on the tops or arms of chairs, knickknacks, photos, books, and plants that adorn the living rooms of most houses not only represent the experiences of a lifetime but also give the environment a rich and varied tactile sense. Some of these familiar objects, such as throw rugs, may be hazardous and therefore are inappropriate in a care setting for frail individuals. However, the sudden change from this tactile-rich setting to one that has almost no variation and includes many hard surfaces is likely to cause some residents to seek sensory stimulation (Figure 4.1).

Other residents may use rummaging as a way of passing time that is otherwise unoccupied. Boredom was addressed in Chapter 2 of this volume, and the same reasons apply to rummaging. Residents who are bored, particularly those who are unable to initiate activity on their own, may rummage through drawers and desks to find something interesting to occupy their attention. When tracking residents' behavior, determine whether rummaging occurs more when there is no ongoing activity on the unit. This is an indication that boredom may be the main cause.

Other residents may rummage because they feel a need to be productive. This is often the case with the person who spends time reorganizing his

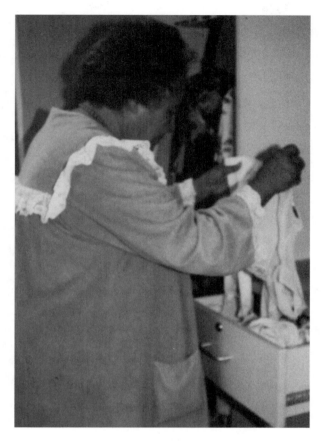

Figure 4.1. Some residents rummage through their own or others' drawers as a means of obtaining sensory stimulation.

or her dresser drawers or closet, or the individual who spends time at the nurses' station gathering papers and sorting through everything. These residents may be trying to be as productive as they used to be but cannot organize their activities enough to be successful.

COMMON REASONS FOR HOARDING

The resident with dementia is experiencing a vast array of losses—memory and cognitive skills, freedom and independence, and social and interpersonal relationships. When it becomes necessary to relocate to a shared residential care setting, these individuals experience the loss of a familiar place and many of their belongings. Hoarding, particularly if the resident carries things around with him or her and is reluctant to give up these items, may be a response to these losses. He or she may be looking for something to hang onto because so much else has been taken away.

Many residents in long-term care lived through the Great Depression of the 1930s. As a consequence, they may have developed a lifelong pattern of saving everything that might conceivably be useful, even that which clearly (at least to others) never will be. This pattern often is manifested in hoarding, whether it is salt, sugar, napkins, or silverware from the dining room; light bulbs from every lamp on the unit; or washcloths out of the clean or soiled linen carts. One clue to understanding what motivates hoarding is where residents put these items. If they try to tuck them away in their drawers or find other hiding spots for them, then a "saving for a rainy day" habit is probably at work. Talking to families may help you learn whether this has been a lifelong pattern, which can be harder to eliminate.

WHAT STAFF CAN DO

Although the reasons for rummaging and hoarding are diverse, there are some relatively simple and common responses that facilities have found useful. Some of these interventions require the facility to alter its philosophy about some issues, especially the tension between ensuring that the unit is tidy for visitors and marketing purposes versus allowing a more cluttered but lived-in look. This is an issue that all levels of staff at the facility need to discuss to arrive at a joint decision about.

Creating Places to Rummage

The most basic and straightforward response to rummaging is to give residents interesting and appropriate places to rummage. Many ideas for creating a rummaging area are described in "What the Environment Can Do." It is also important to determine where these items should be placed. Again, it may depend on the facility's population. Some people may prefer being closer to staff, to be a part of the productive life of the unit. This suggests a location close to the nurses' station or other activity centers. Other residents may prefer to be more secretive about their rummaging and stay in their or other's rooms. Consider providing these "secretive" residents who discretely rummage through others' belongings (which causes problems) with opportunities to rummage in a more remote corner of the unit.

Increasing Sensory Stimulation

Beyond specific places to rummage, staff can consider increasing other sensory stimulation experiences. This can be accomplished in several ways. Ideas for increasing tactile stimulation in the environment in general are provided in "What the Environment Can Do." It is also important to look at the types of activities that are offered. Many of the activities that are commonly offered in long-term care settings provide little in the way of sensory stimulation—particularly softer items. Music can be pleasing, but unless residents are given instruments, it is not a tactile experience. Cooking projects, holiday activities, even seasonal outings can be wonderful opportunities for sensory stimulation and also encourage social interaction.

Providing Opportunities to Be Productive

Some residents rummage or hoard because they feel a need to be productive, so try to redirect them to more appropriate productive activities. Encourage residents to collect items for special projects organized around a theme. The theme could be posted to make it easier to remember. Check with local day care centers or elementary schools to determine whether they are looking for help with special projects in which residents could assist. Another suggestion is to encourage residents to develop collections. This could be as simple as collecting autumn leaves or asking family members to bring in items such as hats, buttons, or old photos from which the residents could choose. You may want to provide space to display these collections, which may serve to limit the size of them, and then use them as part of a special activity.

WHAT THE ENVIRONMENT CAN DO

Often, rummaging is most disruptive when residents take or borrow things from other residents or from staff areas. Their reasons for rummaging may relate to a need for sensory stimulation—particular stimulation that the resident can control and manipulate.

Creating Places to Rummage

When one or more residents routinely engage in rummaging that is disruptive to others, the goal is to redirect the behavior more positively rather than to eliminate the behavior. These residents may be looking for something to do or may be seeking tactile stimulation. To satisfy residents' needs for tactile stimulation, staff should consider providing a variety of accessible, stimulating sensory experiences for residents beyond the regular activities program. Make sure that there are plenty of magazines and coffee table books available to be picked up, looked at, and carried around. Small knickknacks can be added to tabletops and shelves in many of the public areas of the unit. These objects can become the basis of unstructured activities for the residents. Residents who are less able to participate in structured activities may at least enjoy sorting through these objects.

Chests of drawers or boxes filled with a variety of objects with different tactile qualities can be placed in lounges or activity rooms. ("Where to Find Products" at the end of the chapter includes a list of companies that make different types of storage items that can help you create a rummaging area for your residents. Furniture donated by families or purchased at garage sales or flea markets is perfectly acceptable.) Some of the boxes or drawers could be assigned a theme. A sample sewing drawer might include large buttons and beads, yarn, pincushions without pins, and thimbles to sort. Another drawer could contain a collection of miscellaneous hats, from baseball caps to fancy old hats that the women might have worn in their youth. Fill some drawers in the activity room cabinets with napkins, washcloths, or socks to sort and fold.

Encourage residents to handle these objects and to carry the objects around with them. In the beginning, it may be necessary to restock these boxes/chests regularly because some residents may hoard items. Eventually, residents will realize that these are places where one can always find something interesting to touch, look at, or do. Their easily accessible location also makes it easier for staff to provide residents with activities that keep them busy in between structured activity programming. The more accessible that these items are, both to residents who can pick them up independently and to staff to give to less independent residents, the more likely they will be used.

Some facilities create sensory stimulation boards with which residents can tinker. These boards often have various latches, knobs, and other manipulatable items attached. Although such boards may successfully engage some residents' attention, this is not a productive activity, and some residents may perceive this as make-believe or childlike. In general, facilities should try to provide residents with activities that make them feel more productive and are familiar to them.

Creating Places of Productivity

Rummaging at the nurses' station may suggest either an interest in what is going on or a need to continue to feel useful by working. Because many residents worked for most of their adult lives, they may be feeling a lack of productivity. Some high-functioning residents may be looking for activities that provide a sense of accomplishment. Most people have worked at a desk, either in the work or home setting. Try creating a small office area in the corner of the main dining room or lounge, and give residents tasks that need to be done. Setting up the office can be as easy as providing a desk or table. Pens, papers, and files easily can be added by using items found in the facility. Sample tasks for residents who use the desk might include punching holes, stapling, folding newsletters, stamping mail, or rolling coins.

Staff also can re-create many other workplaces for residents to be productive. One facility created a grandmother's corner, with a rocking chair and a small set of shelves that held children's books and soft toys. Visiting families were more comfortable bringing children, knowing that they would have things to play with while on the unit. Men might enjoy baseball cards or other sports memorabilia. One corner of an activity room could be converted into an impromptu workshop. Tools and small machine parts can be placed here—objects that can be screwed in and put together and then taken apart. (Many maintenance departments have an old engine that no longer works that can be cleaned up and offered to the residents.)

Be sure that the activities fit the residents' abilities and interests. These types of tasks do not have to be make-believe but can be of assistance for various everyday events in the facility. Look for ways that residents can help other organizations, so that they can experience the satisfaction of making a real contribution. Many residents could fold flyers for mailing, for instance.

Returning the Idea of Control

Hoarding can be residents' response to feeling a lack of control over their lives. With so much taken away from them over the course of dementia and forced to relocate from home to a care setting, they may be trying to exert some control over something in their lives. Staff may be able to address this need by giving them something to have some control over, such as the items kept in a rummaging drawer. The Eden Alternative philosophy recommends that every resident be given a plant or a bird to care for on admission to alleviate boredom, helplessness, and loneliness (Thomas, 1996).

If the problem seems to be residents wanting to take something from the dining room, staff could consider giving these residents special napkins to take back to their rooms after the meal. These napkins can be ones they have used or napkins for the next meal. Ask them whether they would like to hold onto a napkin until then, and remind them to get their napkins at the next meal. Another suggestion is to give residents a place card with his or her name on it, which could be kept in the resident's room until the next meal.

WHERE TO FIND PRODUCTS

In addition to these sources, check local discount and department stores, the Salvation Army, garage sales, and flea markets for storage units and rummaging items.

Exposures
Post Office Box 3615
Oshkosh, WI 54903-3615
(800) 222-4947
www.exposuresonline.com
A catalog for the storage and display of photographs and mementos.

Hold Everything
Post Office Box 7807
San Francisco, CA 94120-7807
(800) 421-2264
www.holdeverything.com
A catalog of storage items; stores are located in shopping malls across the country (see their website for locations)

JC Penney
(800) 222-6161
Variety of unfinished, easy-to-assemble furniture that can become activity projects for residents

♦ ♦ ♦

A summary sheet follows, which condenses the chapter text into a quick overview. The authors have also provided an area for you to make your own notes about your own staff and facility. Managerial staff may wish to use the summary sheets as handouts to accompany direct care staff training, or to post them by the time clock or nurses' station or include them in staff's pay envelopes.

RUMMAGING AND HOARDING SUMMARY SHEET

1. Recognize that when residents move into a care setting, they are experiencing a series of losses. They may miss having their own personal space filled with their possessions that reflect their personalities. They may miss straightening up and caring for their own homes. They may miss feeling productive.

2. Rummaging can be a positive activity. It provides sensory stimulation and gives residents something interesting to do.

3. Residents rummage in areas where there are things to pick up and sort through. Residents' rooms and the nursing station sometimes look more interesting and inviting than the common spaces. Thus, it is not surprising that residents rummage in these areas.

What Staff Can Do

1. Help each resident to have a sense that they are responsible for something, so that they feel that they have some control over something in their lives. This can be as simple as caring for a plant or animal or holding onto a napkin.

2. Make sure that the common areas contain items that the residents can rummage through, if you do not want residents rummaging in other residents' rooms or staff areas.

3. Set up a specific rummaging area for your residents in a public area. Stock cabinet drawers with a variety of items to sort. You may have to replenish the items or retrieve them from residents' rooms from time to time. These items make great conversation starters and are a source of impromptu activities. Encourage your facility to budget for these items. (If funds are limited, check garage sales or thrift stores or ask for donations of these items from family members.)

4. Offer thematic items that will be of personal interest to the residents who are rummaging. These can be inexpensive, familiar items that relate to residents' past occupations (e.g., a former seamstress may enjoy rummaging through a basket of buttons; a retired mechanic may like handling tool parts, nuts, and bolts). Encourage them to reminisce while rummaging.

5. Assess whether current rummaging presents a real danger for residents. Holding onto a napkin may not pose a problem, whereas hoarding spoiled food poses a health risk.

6. Be creative and devise rummaging activities that are both therapeutic and enjoyable for residents.

7. Try to learn about your residents' past lives from family members to discourage or redirect hoarding. Perhaps saving items has been a lifelong habit of thrift triggered by growing up during or after the Great Depression.

5
Combative Behaviors

Of all of the disruptive behaviors that are exhibited by residents in long-term care facilities, perhaps the most troubling are those that are combative. These behaviors can be physical or verbal and almost always occur in response to something, as discussed in Chapter 1 of this volume. Many times staff are most concerned with physically combative behaviors because of the risk of injury involved. However, verbally combative behaviors should be given equal attention because they can be a precursor to physically combative behavior. Likewise, both types of combative behavior can be triggered by similar interactions or misperceptions. For this reason, the term *combative* in this text refers to both physical and verbal behaviors.

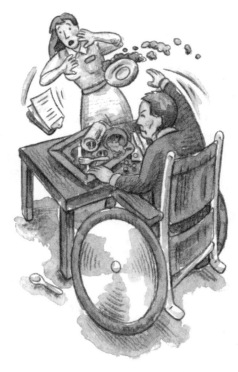

Many facilities report a high occurrence of aggressive behaviors. However, aggressive behaviors as defined in the display on page 76 rarely occur for no reason. In almost all cases something, either an interpersonal interaction or an interpretation of something in the environment, provokes combative behavior, although it can be difficult to identify the "something." Therefore, staff should assume in all cases that something has triggered a resident's combative behavior.

Another term, *resistance to care,* frequently is used to describe one of the most common types of combative behavior. This term is specifically related to residents reacting to staff during personal care. However, because behaviors also can be precipitated by a variety of interactions in addition to personal care. Resistive-to-care behaviors are included under the rubric of *combative behaviors*.

HOW PROBLEMATIC ARE COMBATIVE BEHAVIORS?

Staff of long-term care facilities often view combative behaviors as a major problem on their unit. However, research has found that the frequency of these behaviors often is not as great as some may believe. Studies have found differing results regarding the frequency of combative and argumentative behaviors in long-term care facilities. One study found that frequency of these behaviors varied from one occurrence of a combative behavior every 1½ hours to one occurrence every 5¾ hours (Bridges-Parlet, Knopman, & Thompson, 1994). Despite the relative infrequency of these behaviors, they are likely to be associated with injury and to be a challenge to manage. Therefore, it is not surprising that staff view combative behavior as a serious problem.

When not managed properly, combative behaviors can have a negative impact on all individuals on the unit. Other residents can become frightened, upset, and agitated and may be at risk of injury when they witness combative behaviors. Their reaction may be to act in a similar manner. Staff may become

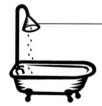

Combative Behaviors Definitions

The literature contains a wide variety of definitions for combative behaviors and what they include. The authors' concept uses the following definitions for various combative behaviors:

- **Physical combativeness** refers to negative physical behaviors that occur in response to specific staff–resident or resident–resident interactions

  Example: A resident strikes out at a staff member who is trying to feed him or her.

- **Verbal combativeness** refers to negative verbal outbursts in response to specific staff–resident or resident–resident interactions.

  Example: A resident yells at a staff member who is undressing him or her.

- **Aggressive behavior** is initiated by the resident and is not obviously a response to a specific interpersonal interaction. Aggressive behaviors can be physical or verbal.

  Example: A resident strikes a person with no apparent provocation.

defensive, irritable, and hurt (physically and emotionally), may blame themselves, or may be unsure of how to react when combative behaviors are aimed at them (Chou, Kaas, & Richie, 1996). The residents who are exhibiting these behaviors are likely to suffer as well. An underlying or unaddressed issue probably caused them to act in this manner in the first place. Unfortunately, staff's response to combative residents is often to avoid them, intentionally or unintentionally. Avoidance can take the form of staff's not completing the intended assistance or passing off the residents' care to another staff member. Either way, the residents' underlying issues or needs may not be addressed.

CAUSES OF COMBATIVE BEHAVIORS

Many people in the field of aging support the belief that, except in rare cases, residents do not act combatively without cause or purpose. For instance, one expert in dementia programs said, "Alzheimer's is a behavioral disease, so when we look at these behaviors, we should not look at them as negatives, but as behavioral symptoms. There is a purpose and meaning behind all behaviors. Our job is to find the purpose" (Gold, 1996, p. 66). There are numerous causes for long-term care residents to react in a combative manner. It is important to determine the cause so that an appropriate intervention can be planned and executed. The different issues that lead to combative behaviors can be divided into three categories: physiological, emotional, and environmental. It is likely that any particular combative episode is a result of issues that fall into two or three of the categories. After reading the description of these types of contributing issues, refer to the case study of Lois in the display below for an example.

Physiological Issues

Physiological issues may be chronic or acute medical or psychiatric conditions. Chronic conditions include organic brain syndrome, bipolar affective disorder, schizophrenia, epilepsy, and temporal lobe abnormalities (Chou et al., 1996). Acute conditions include pain (which the individual may not be able to communicate to staff and which, therefore, has not been adequately treated) and medication imbalances, interactions, or toxicity. Feldt, Warne, and Ryden (1998) examined the possible relationship between pain and aggression in older adults with cognitive impairment using a multifaceted pain assessment. These researchers asked the family members of subjects and the nursing assistants who cared for them whether they thought that residents experienced pain from a physical condition(s); reviewed charts to determine whether subjects had pain-causing medical conditions and if these were being treated with analgesics; and observed the occurrence of aggressive behaviors. They found that 35% of the residents that family members thought were in pain and 56% of the residents that nursing assistants thought were in pain did not receive pain medication. In addition, 60% of the residents who had one

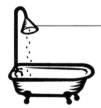

Case Study: Lois

Lois spends a lot of time in her room rearranging her drawers, closet, and nightstand. Unfortunately, the next time she opens her drawers, she has often forgotten that she has rearranged them but does notice that things look different. She assumes someone must have come into her room and gone through her things. Naturally, this is upsetting to her, and she often comes out of her room and yells accusingly at the first person she sees. To that person Lois may appear to be combative without provocation. However, when we look at the situation more closely, we see issues from all three categories (physiological, emotional, and environmental) contributing to Lois' outburst:

- **Physiological:** Memory impairment keeps Lois from remembering that she rearranged her belongings.
- **Emotional:** Seeing her belongings rearranged raises feelings of invasion of personal space, loss of control, and anxiety over who could have done this to her.
- **Environmental:** The change in Lois' physical environment (how she has organized things in her room) contributes to her feelings.

or more pain-causing medical conditions did not receive any pain medication. Significantly higher aggression scores were found in subjects who had two or more pain-causing diagnoses, arthritis, or both. These findings could be explained by the fact that these individuals were experiencing pain associated with movement, so that completion of activities of daily living (ADLs) resulted in their reacting aggressively toward staff who were trying to help them. Thus, whenever combativeness is new in a resident or there is an increase in its occurrence, it is advisable to ask for a physical or psychological assessment or both.

Emotional Issues

Combative behaviors sometimes are related to residents' feelings about a situation. These feelings may include residents' frustration with an inability to communicate to others what they are feeling, a fear of being in unfamiliar surroundings with unfamiliar people, anxiety caused by misinterpreting a given situation, an invasion of their personal space by staff or other residents, or a history of always having acted out their emotions.

Environmental Issues

At times, events occurring on a unit or characteristics of the environment may be disturbing to the resident. Cohen-Mansfield and Werner (1995) found the following environmental conditions to be associated with increased agitation (which can be a precursor to combative behaviors): physical restraints, inactivity, loneliness, decreased staffing levels, and rooms that were cold at night. Other environmental issues that can influence combative behaviors include overstimulation from too much noise or activity on the unit, lack of privacy, disorientation as to where one is, and the mood or attitude expressed by staff or other residents.

The Progressively Lowered Stress Threshold (PLST) model suggests that all individuals can handle only so much stimulation and that if they are overstressed—or get too much stimulation—they can no longer cope (Hall & Buckwalter, 1987). This can help to explain when or why combative behaviors are likely to occur. In general, residents with dementia can tolerate less stimulation than those without dementia, and are therefore more likely to become overwhelmed. The goal in long-term care facilities, then, is to keep residents below their stress threshold. Examples of ways to reduce excess negative stimulation are provided in "What Staff Can Do" and "What the Environment Can Do."

ADDRESSING COMBATIVE BEHAVIORS

Combative episodes directed toward staff often occur during assistance with ADLs. Chou et al. (1996) found that assaultive behavior (their term for various combative behaviors) occurred most frequently during three periods: from 7 A.M. to 10 A.M., from 12 P.M. to 2 P.M., and from 4 P.M. to 7 P.M. Not surprising, these are the times when the majority of ADL assistance occurs (e.g., dressing, bathing, feeding). It is understandable that being on the receiving end of combative behaviors is not a pleasant experience for staff. Reacting with annoyance, frustration, or anger could be seen as natural responses (Gruetzner cited in Potts, Richie, & Kaas, 1996). As a consequence, combative residents' nutritional, toileting, hygiene, and grooming needs may not be met (Potts et al., 1996). Staff must understand that although interacting with combative residents may be stressful, it is necessary if good-quality care is to be provided. This chapter suggests a variety of interventions for preventing and responding to combative behaviors. Because these behaviors are so prevalent during care assistance, it is particularly important to educate direct care staff about the origins of these behaviors and how staff should respond to them. Emphasize to staff that these behaviors rarely are meant as personal attacks at them; rather, such behaviors are the residents' way of expressing an underlying issue (Figure 5.1).

Identifying the Causes

Tracking behaviors is an effective way of finding their patterns and causes. The tracking process involves staff's recording who, what, when, where, and if possible, why a behavior occurred. Implementing a behavior tracking process was discussed in Chapter 1 of this volume. A Behavior Tracking Form that you may wish to copy and use can be found in Appendix A.

If there is no physiological cause for the behavior, then staff should look for possible emotional or environmental causes. One of the best predictors of combative behaviors is a past history of similar behaviors. Thus it is important to talk to the family and friends of a resident about the resident's previous behavior patterns. It is also helpful to find out if there are things that are likely to upset the person (e.g., pet peeves). You may want to consider including this information on the resident's social history forms so that you can anticipate which residents may exhibit these behaviors. Some family members may be reluctant to give you this information or may not be completely honest, either because they are concerned about the repercussions that the dis-

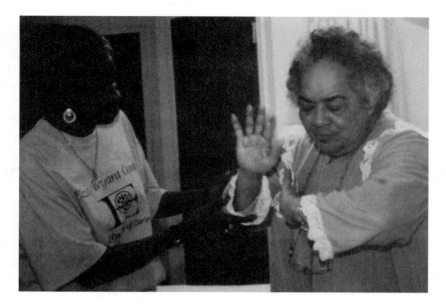

Figure 5.1.   Residents may exhibit combative behavior during assistance with ADLs; staff should not interpret this behavior as a personal attack against them.

closure may have on admission or care provided or they feel embarrassed about it (e.g., the person may have been a verbally abusive spouse or parent).

It is also important to recognize that combative behaviors seldom occur spontaneously. People usually experience a period of buildup until they reach a point at which lashing out seems to be the only or most appropriate way to respond to a given situation. *Buildup* refers to a person's increasing feelings of anxiety, which represent a state of distress or uneasiness. Anxiety is the internal emotion that is usually expressed externally as agitation in the form of general restlessness, pacing, tapping, mumbling, and the like. Staff should learn to recognize the particular levels of agitation of residents who regularly exhibit combative behavior. Learning to look for these cues may make it possible to intervene before the person becomes combative.

Using Restraints

For many years, the most common intervention for combative residents was to restrain them, either physically or with psychotropic medications. Fortunately, this practice is becoming less common. Physical restraints should not be used as an intervention for combative behavior unless a sincere concern for physical harm exists. Furthermore, restraints likely will make a resident even more combative and distressed. (See Chapter 1 of this volume for further discussion on the use of restraints.) "What Staff Can Do" and "What the Environment Can Do" provide a variety of intervention strategies, such as removing excess stimulation, providing quiet time, and allowing residents a sense of control.

Agitation as a Precursor

Because agitation often precedes disruptive behaviors, early intervention at the agitation stage can prevent other, more challenging behaviors. When staff are trained to pay attention to residents' behaviors and moods (this can be a part of the behavior tracking process), they likely will be able to identify agitation that may lead to more explosive behaviors. For example, agitation may be expressed by restlessness, pacing, moaning, or fidgeting. These actions often take the place of a verbal expression that would have been used prior to the onset of dementia. When staff notice these behaviors, they should attempt to talk to the resident about what is bothering him or her or implement an intervention strategy. If combativeness is a serious problem on the unit, or if staff are not responding to agitated behaviors in the preferred manner, then it may be that staff do not understand why residents act this way and are troubled by it. It also may indicate that they have not received adequate training on how to handle these situations.

WHAT STAFF CAN DO

Combative behaviors pose a challenge to long-term care staff. Frequently, staff do not understand the reasons for these behaviors, particularly when a usually calm, polite resident exhibits them. Because there are a wide variety of definitions for these behaviors in the literature, several types of combative behaviors were defined early in the chapter (see the display on p. 76). As discussed there, in almost all cases something provokes the combative behaviors. This section suggests specific social environmental approaches for prevention and intervention.

Staff Training

Thorough, multifaceted staff training is imperative to the success of any long-term care unit or facility. The strategies discussed in this section and in "What the Environment Can Do" all are examples of interventions that either can prevent or reduce combative behaviors. It is extremely important that all staff who interact with residents are trained in the intervention strategies that the facility prefers to use. Certain strategies work better with certain residents. Staff should be encouraged to figure out which strategies work better for specific residents or types of behavior, and these should be part of care planning.

It is also important to inform staff that how they interact with a resident with combative behaviors can affect the success of the intervention. If a resident senses that the staff member is irritated or upset, then he or she may react with increased agitation or combativeness. Staff training also can have an effect on how staff perceive behavior problems. Monahan (1993) used a pretest–posttest research design to assess staff's perceptions. She found that, after staff received training on topics such as cultural and medical perspectives in long-term care and dementia care, Alzheimer's disease, interpersonal relationships, completing ADLs, and adapting activities for residents with dementia, 17 of 36 behaviors on a "Patient Behavior Checklist" were perceived as less problematic at the time of posttest as compared with pretest.

Approaches to Use During Personal Care

One of the most common times that combative behaviors occur is during personal care assistance. Some ideas for preventing the occurrence of these behaviors are provided here.

Dealing with Emotional Issues

It is helpful for staff to try to put themselves in the position of the resident: How would they feel if they needed help being dressed, bathed, or groomed? It is likely that feelings of embarrassment, shame, sadness, and self-consciousness are brought to mind. These are activities that most people have done for themselves for almost their whole lives. It is important for staff to recognize that, even if residents have dementia and do not always seem to be aware of certain things, many still have some of the previously mentioned feelings about needing assistance with care. Furthermore, these residents may not think that they need assistance, or they may not understand that the staff member is only trying to help, and may react to the situation with combative behavior.

Having staff of the same gender assist residents with dressing, bathing, or toileting may help to reduce feelings of self-consciousness. In addition, some residents may have better rapport with certain staff members. Arranging for individual residents' care to be provided by staff with whom they have good relationships whenever possible should help to prevent some episodes of combativeness during care.

Residents may be resistant to undressing during ADLs (or personal care) for a number of reasons. Some residents may feel that undressing in front of someone else is an invasion of their privacy. Others may not understand why staff are asking them to undress or may fear becoming cold. Although some loss of privacy is inevitable when assisting residents with personal care, there are measures that can be taken to minimize this. For example, if the facility has a central or shared tub room, then allow high-functioning residents to choose whether to undress in the tub room or change into a robe in their bedrooms. At all costs, staff should avoid undressing residents in their rooms and simply draping them in a towel or sheet and taking them down the hallway to the tub room.

Using Familiar Routines

Most people have developed routines for when and how they bathe, dress, eat meals, and so forth. Upsetting this routine may cause some residents to become combative. Staff should identify and follow as many of these routines as possible. For instance, find out whether residents usually got dressed before or after breakfast, and what time they usually arose. Getting a habitually late riser out of bed at 6:30 A.M. to go to breakfast is likely to result in agitation, if not combativeness. The facility as a whole must decide what can be done to allow residents' familiar routines to continue. For instance, determine how necessary it is for residents to have breakfast together at the same time, or to eat breakfast at all. If state or federal regulations mandate the minimum and maximum number of hours required between meals, then consider serving a heavy snack late at night to residents who prefer to sleep later than when breakfast is typically served. A continental breakfast could be offered to them when they awaken. Ask the resident's physician how important breakfast is for that resident, and whether an order could be written for breakfast to be skipped if the resident prefers to sleep.

A similar process should be considered for bathing. Whenever possible, staff should make an attempt to allow residents to bathe at a time with which they are comfortable (i.e., morning versus evening). Also allow them the choice of taking a bath or shower. Although these are good approaches to use for all residents (it allows them to make choices, something that is often limited in long-term care), they are especially important for residents who are combative during ADL assistance. Following these residents' previous routines likely will make staff's jobs easier and less stressful as well.

Handling Combativeness During Bathing

Even when residents' prior routines are followed, some residents still are severely upset by taking a bath or shower. Staff should try to find another method of bathing that does not disturb these residents. Other methods to consider include bed baths, sink baths, towel baths, and Comfort Bath or Bag Bath; these methods are described in detail in Volume 2, Chapter 7. "Where to Find Products" at the end of this chapter contains sources for the Comfort Bath and Bag Bath products.

Following residents' preferences or previous bathing routines is ideal, but may not be possible or successful in all cases. Another way to decide how to bathe a resident is to consider the purpose of the bath. Joanne Rader, a geropsychiatric clinical nurse specialist, suggested developing person-focused, individualized bathing care plans by using the three Fs: function, frequency, and form (Hoeffer, Rader, McKenzie, Lavelle, & Stewart, 1997). Once staff determine the function of the bath (e.g., to remove urine, to eliminate body odor) for each resident, then the frequency at which bathing is needed and the form of bathing that is best suited for the function of the bath can be determined.

With the exception of college dormitories, military services, and gym locker rooms, most people are used to bathing privately. Therefore, bathing residents at the same time as other residents or having multiple staff in the room can evoke feelings that are likely to lead to combative behavior. It is important to realize that, although privacy curtains may keep residents from seeing other residents or staff, they do not provide acoustic or olfactory privacy. Noise can be a particular problem because many bathing rooms have hard surfaces that cause noise to reverberate.

Research has found that playing music in the tub room may help reduce agitation and aggression during bathing (Clark, Lipe, & Bilbrey, 1998; Whall et al., 1997). Try to find out what type of music each resident prefers (e.g., classical, hymns, big band). Classical music or nature sounds (e.g., running water in a stream, birds chirping) can be played for residents whose music preference cannot be determined. Whall and colleagues (1997) introduced three "natural elements" to their facility's bathing experience. In addition to playing nature sounds (e.g., bird songs, babbling brooks), they asked the caregivers to show the residents pictures that coordinated with the music being played and try to engage them in conversation during the bath/shower. The third natural element they introduced was food. In their study, they offered residents banana pudding, soda, or both. The food or drink usually was offered during the bathing experience; however, with one resident who was consistently combative during bathing, the researchers first offered the pudding to the resident in her bedroom and told her that she could have more if she came down the hall.

Providing Clear Explanations

Given the verbal/language impairments of some residents with dementia, combativeness during personal care may be a reaction to their inability to understand that staff are trying to assist them. Their combativeness should be viewed as a natural reaction to having something done to them that is typically private. Staff always should talk to residents about the assistance they are providing. Whether residents need cueing or physical assistance, it is important to explain things step by step. Hand gestures or sequencing cards can be helpful for residents with language, hearing, or problem-solving impairments. Sequencing cards can be made or purchased (see "Where to Find Products" for sources). Additional information on the use of sequencing cards is provided in Volume 2, Chapter 6.

Interventions for Overstimulation

Combative behaviors are often the result of an environment that is overstimulating to the resident (refer to the description of the PLST model earlier in this chapter for an explanation). A number of factors can make the environment overstimulating. Several of these factors are dealt with in "What the Environment Can Do," such as noise coming from televisions, radios, public address system(s), or alarms. This section describes people-generated stimulation that staff may be able to change.

Reduce Unnecessary Activity

A lot of non–resident-generated activity can occur on a unit at various times, especially at shift changes, when staff are coming and going. The presence of a number of carts and different types of staff on the unit at the same time also creates traffic and noise, particularly if the unit serves as a pass-through to another unit(s). If possible, a dementia-specific care unit should not be in the path to another part of the facility. This extra traffic can be distracting and upsetting to residents. If this configuration cannot be changed, then try to alter the schedule so that at least carts and other equipment only go through at times when residents will be less likely to notice them. It is best to distribute the passage of carts and equipment across the day, so that there are no periods of excessive traffic. Another option is to arrange to have the carts come on the unit when most residents are involved in an activity, such as being in the dining room for a meal. Because it may be harder to schedule when people move through the unit, the facility should develop a policy to encourage people to be as quiet and unobtrusive as possible when passing through.

Incorporate Quiet Times

Incorporating regularly scheduled quiet times into the daily program can occur on an individual basis in bedrooms or with quiet, calm music in a small social space. Tracking combative behavior may reveal specific times when one or more residents are combative. Scheduling a quiet time for 30–45 minutes before these intervals can help to alleviate any anxiety or agitation that may lead to combativeness.

Intervening in a Combative Situation

Despite the best efforts of staff to prevent combative situations, they will still occur from time to time. All staff of a facility need to know how to respond to a combative resident. When the resident is in a room with other residents, staff should either remove the upset resident or remove the other residents. It is sometimes easier to ask the other residents to leave the room if the upset resident is reluctant to listen to you. In addition, it is likely that the outburst will upset the other residents, and they may be anxious to get away from the combative resident. If a resident becomes upset with a staff member (e.g., when he or she tries to help the resident), it may be best for that staff member to leave the resident alone for a time. This allows the resident to calm down and gives the staff member the chance to think of a new approach. After some time has passed, the staff member, or another person who has a good rapport with the resident, can approach the resident again.

It is important to be aware of how to approach a resident who is exhibiting combative behavior. Residents can pick up on staff's attitude or mood through their tone of voice and body language. If a resident senses that you are irritated or upset, then he or she may react by becoming more combative. Staff should approach the resident slowly, announce who they are, try to gain eye contact, and get the resident's attention by gently stroking or holding his or her hand (Evans, 1991). Be calm and reassuring until you are sure that the resident has calmed down. If the resident is really upset, then it may take awhile for him or her to calm down. Try to talk to the resident and find out what is bothering him or her. It is especially important to talk to family members of residents with diminished communication skills about things that might be upsetting to these residents. Staff also should spend more time unobtrusively observing these residents to identify events or people that set off combative behaviors.

WHAT THE ENVIRONMENT CAN DO

The previous sections of this chapter described a variety of reasons why residents may become combative. Once again, staff should remember that there is almost always a cause for combative behavior, and the best way to avoid its occurrence—and the potential negative consequences of it—is to figure out why the resident is combative and address that underlying concern. This section describes some ways the physical environment can be modified to deal with combativeness.

Addressing Combative Behaviors During Bathing

Hand-Held Shower Wands

Some residents may become combative in the shower either because the water spraying from the showerhead frightens them or because they do not have control over the stream of water hitting them. For example, depending on their height, or if they are sitting in a shower chair, the stream of water may hit them in the face or make their hair wet, which may upset them. Hand-held shower wands can alleviate this problem because they allow the water flow to be controlled (Figure 5.2). Facilities that have not installed hand-held shower wands should do so in all showers and tubs. Encourage staff to adjust the height or direction of the shower head for different residents. Some residents may prefer to hold, or have staff hold, the shower wand in their hand. This allows them to wash and rinse different parts of their bodies individually.

Bathtubs that Fit Residents' Needs

Some residents may become upset during bathing because of the unfamiliarity of many institutional tubs. The tub may look or feel different, causing them to not understand what it is or be fearful of what is going to happen to them. By using a sensitive and compassionate approach toward residents, staff can

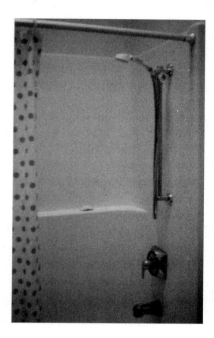

Figure 5.2. Hand-held shower wands provide residents with more control over the water and can reduce combative behavior during bathing.

alleviate some of their anxiety. Other considerations regarding bathtubs can make a difference in preventing combative behavior (Table 5.1). A tub that can be filled before the resident enters it and that does not require a chair lift can be helpful with high-functioning residents. Residents with significant impairment should be bathed in tubs that accommodate both seated and supine bathing. Whenever possible, avoid using tubs that require a resident to be lifted high off the ground. (See "Where to Find Products" for sources of various tubs and showers.)

Respecting Privacy

Some residents are combative because they do not like to be nude in front of "strangers" (including familiar staff). Several nurses have told the authors that keeping the resident covered with a sheet and washing under the sheet does a remarkable job at eliminating combativeness. This works in both showers and tubs. Also, a half-height shower curtain can be hung across the shower opening to provide some privacy for residents and help keep caregivers dry (see "Where to Find Products" for sources).

Table 5.1.   Comparison of bathing tub models

	Side-entry tilting tubs	Front-entry tubs	Side-entry tubs with door	Lift-over tubs
Use	Lift-up side doors and a pre-filled water footwell; once resident has entered the tub, tub tilts back and water from the footwell fills remainder of tub	Front-entry door that works well with special chairs or lifts that glide resident back into bathing areas; prefilled chamber fills tub with temperature-adjusted water in 90 seconds after door is shut	Side-entry doors with built-in seats; doors may swing out, roll down or swing up, depending on model; tub fills with temperature-adjusted water after door is shut	These tubs require a resident be lifted over to enter it; tub can be raised or lowered to aid the caregiver
Options and features	Companion lifts Adjustable heights Remote locatable controls Electric tilt Hand-held shower wand	Companion carrier Available with UV light (eliminates bacteria) Hand-held shower wands	Companion lifts Can be mounted in a recess similar to a residential tub Hand-held shower wands	Companion lifts Some models can be raised and lowered
Pros	Emulates actual bathing by allowing bather to adjust to water temperature before being immersed in water Controls can be located behind a curtain to lessen institutional appearance Side entry allows for easy transfer of ambulatory residents Whole body of resident easily reachable by caregiver	Offers quick bathing with 90-second fill and quick drain Tub temperature and water level controlled by the tub once set rather than staff monitoring Tub allows for fairly easy transfer of nonambulatory residents into tub	With built-in appearance on some models it can resemble a residential tub Side-entry door provides dignified entry for ambulatory residents Some models allow for resident to bathe unassisted	Some units allow supine bathing Can use a standard residential tub in a recessed platform for a residential appearance

Cons	Tilting of tub may disorient some residents Tub has an institutional appearance Motion of some manual hydraulic models may be jerky Because of how it operates, tub must be used with assistance	Quick water fill from behind may disturb some residents Tub has an institutional appearance Some residents may not like cold room temperature while waiting for tub to fill Ambulatory residents still must use transfer chair and be assisted when bathing Feet of resident are positioned low and hard to reach	Nonresidential controls may confuse/disturb residents Some seats are too upright and use straps to keep residents from slouching Some large doors are difficult to operate and may pinch residents Some residents may not like cold room temperature while waiting for tub to fill	Lift-over chairs can be frightening for resident and difficult for staff to use Companion lifts are only way to easily transfer a resident who is unable to step over tub Low tubs may be difficult for caregiver to use Some models can be very institutional in appearance
Sources	Arjo, Inc., 50 North Gary Avenue Roselle, IL 60172 (800) 323-1245 *www.arjo.com*	Apollo Post Office Box 219 450 Main Street Somerset, WI 54025 (800) 247-5490 (715) 247-5625 *www.apollobath.com*	Apollo Post Office Box 219 450 Main Street Somerset, WI 54025 (800) 247-5490 (715) 247-5625 *www.apollobath.com* Arjo, Inc., 50 North Gary Avenue Roselle, IL 60172 (800) 323-1245 *www.arjo.com* Invacare 739 Goddard Avenue Chesterfield, MO 63005 (800) 347-5440 *www.invacare-ccg.com*	Arjo, Inc., 50 North Gary Avenue Roselle, IL 60172 (800) 323-1245 *www.arjo.com* Invacare 739 Goddard Avenue Chesterfield, MO 63005 (800) 347-5440 *www.invacare-ccg.com*

Creating Pleasant Tub Rooms

Most tub rooms are filled with hard, antiseptic-looking surfaces. Although tile wall surfaces may be necessary for cleanliness, they do not create a calm and pleasant atmosphere. Bathrooms are often noisy rooms, and some people are sensitive to this noise. Tub rooms also look very foreign and institutional. To provide visual interest, consider adding a few plants or artwork or colorful towels and privacy curtains. Try to create a grooming area with a vanity, seat, and mirror. This might be as easy as providing a table with a skirt and a mirror hung above it (Figure 5.3). A large flower arrangement on this vanity can make the room seem friendly. A more soothing acoustical environment might be achieved by playing soft or preferred music to calm agitated residents. Moisture-proof acoustical panels also can be used to reduce some of the noise in these rooms (see "Where to Find Products" for sources). These panels can be adhered to ceilings or walls that are located out of the splash zone.

Pleasant rather than antiseptic smells also contribute to an improved environment. One facility has found that aromatherapy has calmed residents. This can be as simple as adding a few drops of lavender-scented oil on a light bulb in the room. Aromatherapy diffusers are commercially available in many department stores, and plug-in room fresheners can be used as well. (See "Where to Find Products" for sources of aromatherapy products.) Some residents may resist bathing in the tub room because it is too cold. Heat lamps or radiant heat panels can provide supplemental heat to make the room more comfortable. Playing soft, pleasant music in the tub room also may help to create a pleasant environment and reduce anxiety and agitation during bathing.

Addressing Environmental Auditory and Visual Causes of Stress

Noise Reduction

Excess stimulation on the unit also can lead to combativeness. If a behavior tracking evaluation indicates that residents are often combative when the unit is noisy or chaotic, then try a stimulation assessment. The Sensory Stimulation Assessment form found in Appendix B can be used to isolate the various sources of stimulation. When residents are agitated or combative, record what is occurring on the unit on the form. Use this information to minimize any traffic through the unit, reschedule carts and other potentially distracting support services, and eliminate or minimize other sources of stimulation. If combativeness seems to coincide with television or radio news programming, then turn off the television and radios at these times.

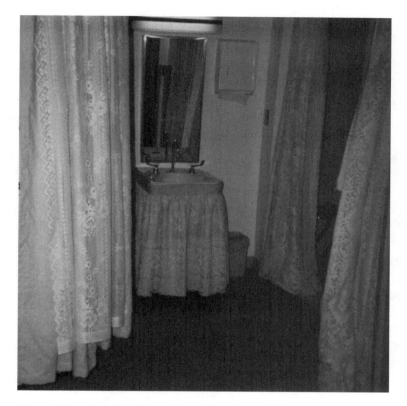

Figure 5.3.   A vanity with a mirror above it can help to make the bathroom more pleasant.

Staff should be aware that noise—particularly unpredictable noises such as call bells and alarms—can increase agitation in many residents. A number of call bell systems use staff pagers and are not as noisy. Sources for these systems are included in "Where to Find Products" at the end of this chapter. Although call bell usage cannot be controlled, staff should try to answer the bells immediately so that they can be turned off.

Another source of noise that can cause agitation among residents with dementia is the public address system. Ideally, the facility should eliminate this system altogether on units with residents with dementia. Consider asking key staff to wear beepers, which generate significantly less noise than public address systems. Technology has advanced such that every staff member can have his or her own combined beeper and cellular phone. This system not only provides silent paging for staff but also has instant two-way communication capabilities. If installation of such a system is not possible, then try to limit the use of the public address system so that there are periods of quiet or that it is only used for emergencies.

Appropriate Television and Music Programming

Many people with dementia find it difficult to separate what they see on television from their own lives. Therefore, staff should monitor the programs to which residents with dementia are exposed. Talk shows, news programs, police shows, and soap operas can be disturbing and may foster delusions and paranoia. Game shows and cartoons also can be disturbing to residents because of their frequent shifts in mood and background music. If some residents enjoy these shows and are not negatively affected by them, then staff can determine whether these shows can be played in a noncentralized area of the unit, and can keep residents who are disturbed by them (or any agitated resident) away from the television. Conversely, television can aid in soothing residents who are agitated. Videos of nature or animals may calm residents. Showing movies from residents' youth (1930s–1950s), especially musicals, often can keep residents with dementia content.

Likewise, staff should pay attention to what types of music are being played for residents because some types may lead to combative behaviors, whereas others can have a calming effect or bring on reminiscence. For example, staff may consider light rock acceptable because it sounds rather calm and pleasant as compared with classical or hard rock music. However, even if staff think such music sounds soothing, residents are unlikely to be familiar with contemporary songs. In addition, although some radio stations play "soft" music, others lean toward rock, which typically places emphasis on the second beat of the music. Residents in long-term care facilities belong to a generation that is used to music in which the emphasis is on the first beat, and thus may find listening to rock, even soft rock, disturbing. Finally, Muzak is intentionally programmed to encourage more movement and activity, along with periods of quieter, more relaxing music. This may or may not match resident scheduling in the facility and probably should be avoided.

The volume of the television or music also can have an impact on residents' behaviors. Music that is too loud or the presence of other noise in the background may be overstimulating for some residents. Admittedly, finding the right volume level can be tricky. Residents may have varying degrees of hearing impairment. When music is used in an activity or program, residents with the most severe hearing impairment should sit closest to the source of music.

Despite these concerns, music can be a powerful source of positive stimulation and enjoyment. Appropriate types of music to play include classical, oldies, religious/gospel, or appropriate ethnic (e.g., polka, English brass band) music. In some regions, residents may prefer country music. Staff should try to determine what type of music residents are accustomed to hearing. When music is used as an individual activity, headphones prevent the music from disturbing other residents. Some residents may not like headphones or may take time to get used to them, but staff should be patient and keep trying. Headphones can be effective because they block out conflicting noises.

Acoustical Treatments

Sound-absorbing materials can be added on noisy units. Facilities that already have acoustical tiles in the ceiling can hang acoustical wall products on the lower portion of the walls to reduce noise as well as protect the walls from damage from wheelchairs and carts. Several wall coverings also are available that help reduce noise reverberation to some degree. Information on locating these panels and wall coverings is provided in "Where to Find Products."

Glare Reduction

As people age, it takes longer to adjust to changes in light levels. During this adaptation period, a person may be functionally blind or unable to see clearly, which could lead to combativeness in some residents. In addition, residents' eyes constantly are adjusting in a unit where there is a lot of glare, which can be tiring. Accordingly, staff should try to reduce glare throughout the unit. The type of glare must be determined, and there are two broad categories of glare: direct glare from an unshielded light bulb or direct sunlight coming in windows, and indirect glare reflected off a surface, such as sunlight on a shiny floor. Windows and the areas around windows are often places with glare.

When the facility is selecting window coverings, some means of filtering the incoming light should be provided. Metal or plastic vertical and horizontal blinds are not the best choice because they create alternating slits of light and dark that can be disorienting to residents with dementia. In addition, light can reflect off metal blinds, causing even more glare. Window treatments that allow light to be diffused without totally blocking the view are preferable. One way to achieve this is with a combination of sheers and drapes. Fabric horizontal blinds and shades made of translucent material that prevents glare while allowing filtered light through also work nicely.

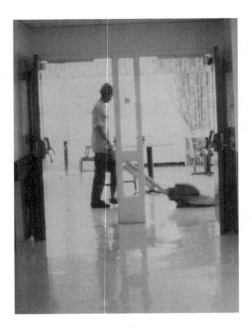

Figure 5.4.   Polishing floors to a high gloss
can cause indirect glare from reflected sunlight, which can confuse or temporarily blind
residents and lead to combative behavior.

Shiny, clean floors are another source of indirect glare (Figure 5.4).
However, "clean" does not have to mean "shiny." Instead of polishing floors,
considering buffing them with a cleanser that provides a matte finish. Administrators may be concerned that families will be upset when they try this,
thinking the facility is not as clean as it was the last time they visited. Administrators may want to write letters to family members explaining that the
facility is purposefully eliminating the shine because the indirect glare is det-
rimental to residents' well-being.

Another common source of glare is lighting, particularly in hallways.
Lights that shine directly down create pools of light on polished floors. This
is particularly hazardous because these pools of light move when residents
walk. They easily can be misinterpreted as pools of water on the floor, causing
residents to try to walk around or step over them, increasing the risk of falls.
Although changing the lighting can be an expensive modification, facilities
that are considering new lighting should look into using indirect lights that
reflect the light up onto the ceiling (if the ceiling is high enough) or down

the hallway walls, decreasing reflective glare on the floor. The use of carpeting also eliminates glare that is reflected from a floor. (See "Where to Find Products" for sources of lighting and lighting consultants.)

Mirrors

Care should be taken when using mirrors in a dementia-specific unit because they can be a source of agitation for some residents. For example, if a resident with dementia sees his or her reflection in a mirror while walking into the bathroom, then he or she may think the room is occupied. Walls made of mirrors may be disorienting to residents with dementia. Some may become agitated thinking that a similar-looking relative is coming to see them when they see their own reflection. Conversely, other residents experience a calming effect when talking with their reflection. The best practice is to use mirrors in places where they are normally located. Staff who believe that mirrors are a source of agitation for a particular resident should look for ways to remove the mirror or cover the surface. Also, uncovered windows become reflective at night in brightly lit rooms. Residents may misinterpret images that are reflected and become agitated or combative. Window coverings that block this illusion are an easy solution to this problem.

WHERE TO FIND PRODUCTS

Alternative Bathing Products

Incline Technologies
(800) 538-0205
www.inclinetechnologies.com
Manufactures Bag Bath, a prepackaged disposable bathing system; moistened cloths containing a quick-evaporating cleansing solution

Sage Products, Inc.
3909 Three Oaks Road
Gary, IL 60013
(800) 323-2220
www.sageproducts.com
Comfort Bath, a prepackaged system of eight disposable washcloths that can be heated in a microwave

Sequencing Cards

AliMed, Inc.
297 High Street
Dedham, MA 02026
(800) 225-2610
www.alimed.com

Communication Skill Builders/Therapy Skill Builders
Post Office Box 839954
San Antonio, TX 78283-3954
(800) 211-8378
www.hbem.com; *www.psychcorp.com*

Imaginart
307 Arizona Street
Bisbee, AZ 85603
(800) 828-1376
e-mail: imaginart@aol.com
Pick 'n Stick communication products

Mayer-Johnson, Inc.
Post Office Box 1597
Solana Beach, CA 92075
(800) 588-4548
www.mayer-johnson.com
Boardmaker and Board Builder

Tubs and Showers

Apollo Corporation
Post Office Box 219
Somerset, WI 54025
(800) 247-5490
www.apollobath.com

Aquarius Bathware LLC
Praxis Industries, Inc.
435 Industrial Road
Savannah, TN 38372
(800) 443-7269
www.aquariusproducts.com
Tub with extra-large grab bars

Arjo, Inc.
50 North Gary Avenue, Unit A
Roselle, IL 60172
(800) 323-1245
www.arjo.com

BathEase
3815 Darston Street
Palm Harbor, FL 34658
(727) 786-2604

Comfort Designs
Post Office Box 34279
Richmond, VA 23234
(800) 801-2820

Edison Lyle
Post Office Box 728
Jonesboro, GA 30237
(800) 444-0888
Manufactures Freedom Bath

Invacare
528 Hughes Drive
Traverse City, MI 49683
(800) 347-5440
www.invacare-ccg.com

Sunrise Medical
5001 Joerns Drive
Stevens Point, WI 54481
(800) 826-0270
www.sunrisemedical.com

Half-Height Shower Curtains

Invacare
528 Hughes Drive
Traverse City, MI 49683
(800) 678-7100
www.invacare-ccg.com

Acoustical Treatments

Conwed Designscape
800 Gustafson Road
Ladysmith, WI 54848
(800) 932-2383
www.conweddesignscape.com

Illbruck Architectural Products
3800 Washington Avenue North
Minneapolis, MN 55412
(800) 225-1920
www.illbruck-archprod.com
Contour and Squareline acoustical panels with stain-resistant surfaces

JM Lynne Co., Inc.
59 Gilpin Avenue
Post Office Box 1010
Smithtown, NY 11787
(800) 645-5044
www.jmlynne.com
Flame-retardant acoustical textile wallcoverings

Pyrok, Inc.
1313 Bustling Lane
Marietta, GA 30064
(404) 607-9765
www.buildingmaterialsdir.com
Durable, paintable acoustical plaster

Silent Paging Systems

Alarmtec Systems
120 Brookswood
Sherwood, AR 72120
(501) 839-2079
www.alarmtec.com

Cornell Communications
1640 West Silver Spring Drive
Milwaukee, WI 53209
(800) 558-8957
www.cornell.com

JTECH Communications, Inc.
6413 Congress Avenue, Suite 150
Boca Raton, FL 33487
(800) 321-6221
www.jtech.com
PeopleAlert Messaging System, a silent nurses' call system

Spectralink
5755 Central Avenue
Boulder, CO 80301
(800) 676-5485
www.spectralink.com

Worldwide Timing Systems, Inc.
4974 Provident Drive
Cincinnati, OH 45246
(800) 543-7441
www.wwtsinc.com
Voice call and Night-n-gale wireless communication systems

Lighting

Lighting Consultants

Eunice Noell-Waggoner
Center for Design for an Aging Society
6200 Southwest Virginia Avenue, Suite 210
Portland, OR 97201
(503) 246-8231
Noell-Waggoner is an expert in the field of lighting for aging people.

Illuminating Engineering Society of North America (IESNA)
120 Wall Street, Floor 17
New York, NY 10005
(212) 248-5000
www.iesna.org
Lighting and the Visual Environment for Senior Living (1998)

Lighthouse International
111 East 59th Street
New York, NY 10022-1202
(800) 829-0500
www.lighthouse.org
Offers a variety of solutions and products for individuals with visual impairment

Architectural Lighting Systems
30 Sherwood Drive
Taunton, MA 02780
(508) 823-8277
Cove lighting

Holophane Co.
214 Oakwood Avenue
Newark, OH 43055
Baffles for fluorescent lights

Microsun, Inc.
(800) 657-0077
www.microsun.com
Floor and table lamps that use combination incandescent and metal halide lamps to provide high-efficiency, high-level lighting

Schumaker Lighting, Inc.
Adjustable Fixture Co.
3726 North Booth Street
Milwaukee, WI 53223-4714
(800) 558-2628
www.adjustablefixture.com

SPI Lighting Inc.
10400 North Enterprise Drive
Mequon, WI 53092
(414) 242-1420
www.spilighting.com
Phaces wall scones that meet the 4-inch clearance standard and come with a variety of lighting options

Aromatherapy

Gaiam
(formerly Selfcare)
360 Interlocken Boulevard, Suite 300
Broomfield, CO 80021-3440
(877) 989-6321
www.gaiam.com

Heat Lamps

Nu-Tone
Madison and Red Bank Roads
Cincinnati, OH 45227-1599
(800) 543-8687

♦ ♦ ♦

A summary sheet follows, which condenses the chapter text into a quick overview. The authors have also provided an area for you to make your own notes about your own staff and facility. Managerial staff may wish to use the summary sheets as handouts to accompany direct care staff training, or to post them by the time clock or nurses' station or include them in staff's pay envelopes.

COMBATIVE BEHAVIORS SUMMARY SHEET

1. Combativeness refers to negative physical behaviors occurring in response to specific staff to resident or resident to resident interactions.

2. Combat combativeness:

    C = Consider when these behaviors occur. Look for clues that indicate that a resident is becoming upset, and intervene before the resident becomes combative.

    O = Offer an explanation before providing personal care. Combative behaviors often occur because residents do not understand what a staff member is trying to do with or to them. Always explain what you are doing and why to residents. Use simple language and hand gestures to demonstrate. Always perform personal care in a quiet, private space. Put yourself in the resident's shoes and imagine how you would feel if someone was trying to undress or bathe you. Remember that a single staff member's approaching the resident to provide care is less threatening than are multiple staff members.

    M = Minimize conflict. Determine what is making the resident agitated and remove or eliminate it. If other residents are present, either separate the upset resident or direct other residents away from the combative incident.

    B = Be flexible. If a resident is upset with you, back off and give him or her some time to cool off. Then reapproach him or her in a calm, slow manner. Ask another staff member to take your place if you think that the resident may still be upset with you.

    A = Make appropriate television program and music choices. Show old movies that are familiar to the residents. Show nature programs, which can have a calming effect on residents. Play music that your residents are familiar with, such as classical, oldies, and ethnic music (e.g., polkas). Schedule times when televisions/radios are turned off. Do not show soap operas, news programs, or talk shows to residents who tend to be combative. These shows frequently have disturbing content, and people with dementia may have a hard time separating television from reality. Do not play contemporary music, including light rock—your residents probably are not familiar with this music.

    T = Do not allow too much noise on the unit. Noise and commotion can overwhelm residents with dementia, causing them to become combative. Limit the use of the public address system; use it only for emergencies, not just for staff's convenience. Turn call bells and alarms off as soon as possible. Do not play the television and radio at the same time if they are near each other. Provide a quiet space for residents to sit without televisions and radios playing.

6

Socially Inappropriate Behaviors

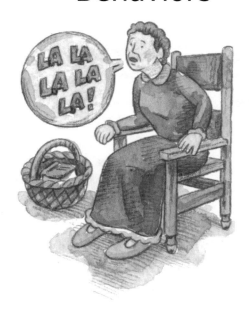

The term *disruptive vocalizations* refers to noises made by residents that can be intermittent or continuous, with or without purpose, varying in level of loudness, and understandable or unintelligible (Ryan, Tainsh, Kolodny, Lendrum, & Fisher, 1988). For example, some residents may scream or call out for attention with a specific purpose, such as expressing that they are thirsty or need to use the bathroom. Others may moan in unintelligible sounds for extended periods of time. Disruptive vocalizations have been found to occur in 25%–30% of residents of long-term care facilities (Cohen-Mansfield, Werner, & Marx, 1990; Ryan et al., 1988). Residents who exhibit such behavior frequently have late-stage dementia. These residents may use a limited number of words, may need extensive assistance with activities of daily living (ADLs), and may have hearing or vision impairments.

Contributing Factors

Although it may appear as if some residents with advanced dementia exhibit this behavior without purpose, there is almost always some reason for the behavior. Disruptive vocalizations may be an expression of feelings of agitation, or residents may simply mimic the actions or moods of others (White, Kaas, & Richie, 1996). If a resident interprets a caregiver's mood as irritated or upset,

Table 6.1. Disruptive vocalizations: Causes and contributing factors

Type	Possible cause	Contributing factors
"Leave me alone!"	Environmental overstimulation	Excess noise, glare, or traffic on unit
Moaning	Pain, discomfort	Untreated medical condition; need for repositioning
"Nurse, nurse!"	Understimulation, often a result of immobililty or restrictions of freedom	Physical restraints or being bedbound keep these residents from being able to provide themselves with stimulation.
"Na, na, na . . ." (perseverative)	Sensory impairment	No appropriate sensory stimulation for low-functioning residents
"Help me!" "Oh, God!"	Depression, anxiety, loneliness	Calls for help or attention
"No! No!"	Misinterpretation of caregiver behavior	Caregiver attempts to help resident undress
Swearing	Lowered inhibitions	Anything that might cause a person to swear

then the resident may respond with vocally disruptive behavior. Table 6.1 lists types of vocalizations, potential or possible causes for them, and environmental factors that may contribute to the vocalizations (Sloane, 1996).

Assessing Behavior

The best way to assess this behavior is to use a multidisciplinary team whose various types of training may elicit different observations. One research study suggested using the following steps to gather information to develop a treatment plan (Sloane, 1996):

1. Describe the resident's behavior.
2. Listen to the message or meaning being expressed.
3. Determine what triggers the behavior.
4. Assess the cognitive and physical status of the resident.
5. Ask family members about any past events or history of depression or other psychiatric disorders that may be contributing to the behavior.

6. Identify what relieves the vocalizations. You may want to ask family members or friends about types of positive stimulation from which the resident may benefit. (Examples of interventions are provided in "What Staff Can Do.")
7. Use the information gathered from the previous steps to develop a management plan. Inform all staff about this plan.

Discussing the Behavior with Direct Care Staff

Inform direct care staff about the possible causes and contributing factors of vocally disruptive behaviors. As a result of the disruptiveness and social inappropriateness of these behaviors, staff may be inclined to think of vocally disruptive residents as demanding or grumpy. Help them to understand that the vocalizer likely is suffering from or in need of something and is not behaving this way to be spiteful or demanding.

It is particularly important to emphasize to direct care staff that a resident's vocalization may be an indication of pain or discomfort, especially if the resident is moaning. Tell staff that this behavior should be brought to the attention of the charge nurse. It is possible that the resident has a PRN (as needed) order for pain medication. Likewise, inform them that more frequent repositioning may alleviate the pain and discomfort often felt by immobile residents.

Finally, staff should be aware of how their actions can affect this behavior. Calling out across the unit to one another and to other residents can be a source of excess stimulation that can lead to expressions of disruptive behaviors, as can overuse of the public address system or television. The manner in which staff approach residents can affect how residents will respond. General suggestions for staff include approaching slowly; using a calm, unrushed voice; making eye contact with the resident; and explaining any actions or assistance they plan to give before doing so.

INAPPROPRIATE SEXUAL BEHAVIORS

Occasionally, residents with dementia engage in sexual behaviors. Although this type of behavior may not be observed as frequently as other behaviors (e.g., wandering, combativeness), it can be one of the most difficult for staff to address. These behaviors include masturbating, talking in suggestive ways, touching or grabbing at staff or other residents, kissing and holding hands with another individual, and engaging in sex. Although these behaviors are varied, they can be disturbing to staff, residents, and visitors. Staff may not know how to respond to the resident(s) or may have conflicting opinions about what residents should and should not do. Therefore, this issue should not be ignored but rather discussed openly, and a protocol should be in place so that staff know how to respond to residents' sexual behaviors. It is also important to have open dialogues with incoming residents and their families so that they are aware of the facility's policies and can share their own desires regarding these issues. The following text defines and discusses the different types of sexual behaviors and issues that should be considered. "What Staff Can Do" addresses planning protocols for responding to the behaviors, including how to determine the informed consent of residents engaging in sexual behaviors and how to work with family members.

Resident Sexuality

A number of sexual behaviors may be seen in a facility. These behaviors can be divided into three categories. First, some residents have a spouse or significant other (who may or may not be living in the facility) and wish to continue to have sexual or intimate contact with him or her. Second, relationships can form between residents of the facility. Third, residents may masturbate, disrobe in public, touch or grab at others, and make verbal advances toward others. The latter category consists of behaviors that are most commonly considered *inappropriate sexual behavior.* Each of these categories is addressed separately.

There is a common misperception that older adults have no interest in engaging in sexual or intimate relationships. However, sexuality and intimacy are important aspects of many people's lives across the life span. Many older adults who are active and physically able remain sexually active. When older adults begin to need help with self-care activities and can no longer live independently, people have a tendency to not consider their sexual or intimacy needs. Having dementia does not make these desires or needs go away. Neither does living in a long-term care facility. These two situations do complicate matters, though. Thus, it is not surprising that this is an issue in many long-term care settings, despite the fact that it is seldom discussed in public.

The importance of intimacy and sexual relationships vary with every resident. For some residents with spouses or significant others, engaging in sex may have become less important than maintaining an enduring emotional attachment. For other couples, sex continues to be an important component of their relationship. Either way, couples have the right to demand some privacy during their visits, regardless of whether they want to have a private conversation and hold hands or be more intimate.

Some residents may form relationships with other residents. Often, these relationships are a source of companionship and may never go beyond holding hands. Others may wish to engage in sexually intimate behaviors, including intercourse. If two residents become attracted to each other, are not married, and are mentally competent, then it is hard to justify trying to keep them apart, except perhaps when there are medical contraindications. Challenges arise, however, when the individuals are married or when one or both have dementia.

Inappropriate sexual behaviors include masturbating (particularly in public), disrobing in public, touching or grabbing at others, and making verbal advances toward others. You may or may not view these behaviors as inappropriate; they are labeled as such for categorization purposes. In many cases, the context in which the behavior occurs determines whether the behavior is appropriate or inappropriate. Likewise, individual beliefs and viewpoints influence how these behaviors are viewed. Some of these behaviors are considered inappropriate because they take place in public and may be offensive to others. Typically, these residents do not mean to be offensive, but they have lost their concept of what constitutes appropriate behavior in public. This loss of inhibitions and inability to follow social conventions is a common consequence of progressive dementia and can be difficult to manage. Other behaviors are considered inappropriate because of the individual(s) toward whom they are displayed. For example, it is generally inappropriate to grab at or make explicit verbal sexual advances toward anyone. More subtle advances, such as asking for a date or a kiss, may also be considered inappropriate by some staff and residents.

Underlying Causes

Need for Affection and Intimacy

Wanting and seeking affection is a normal human behavior that may be the underlying cause of many sexual behaviors (whether considered inappropriate or appropriate). The male resident who makes sexual advances daily toward the nurses and nursing assistants simply may be seeking personalized nonsexual attention. Some residents may turn to other residents when they are looking for affection or attention. Residents who were accustomed to living with a spouse or significant other may miss the hugs, kisses, and companionship they used to enjoy. When residents seek affection from others, it is possible that their behavior will escalate beyond simple hand holding and conversation. Sometimes, staff may intervene in fear of what *may* happen next, when in fact it never would have progressed beyond holding hands.

Forgetting What Is Appropriate Behavior

Sometimes, residents with dementia may forget what is appropriate in particular situations. For example, when a resident undresses or disrobes in public, which is sometimes considered a sexually inappropriate behavior, it is often an attempt to express a different need. The resident may have gotten overheated in his or her clothing, may need to go to the bathroom, or may simply feel uncomfortable. A male resident may walk around with his genitals exposed because of an open zipper, which may happen simply because the resident did not complete the task of dressing or forgot to zip his zipper after urinating. Zeiss, Davies, and Tinklenberg (1996) categorized this type of behavior as *sexually ambiguous behavior* instead of *sexually inappropriate behavior* because it does not necessarily consist of an overt act with sexual meaning.

Medical or Physical Causes

When a resident is masturbating or touching him- or herself, staff should recognize that this may not be done purely for sexual pleasure. It is important to rule out possible medical conditions. Men may be suffering from a urinary tract infection, scabies, or a skin rash (Hellen, 1995; Philo, Richie, & Kaas, 1996). Medical conditions that may be present in women include urinary tract infection, vaginitis, prolapsed uterus, labial cancer, or skin rashes. Also, neurological changes in the brain of a person with dementia may cause a decrease in impulse control (Philo et al., 1996). This decreased impulse control can influence a variety of behaviors, such as making sexual advances or masturbating in public.

REPETITIVE BEHAVIORS

Another behavior that some people believe to be inappropriate is *repetitive behavior*, also known as perseverance. This includes both repetitive movements and vocalizations. Some of these behaviors are harmless, but some can be either harmful to the individual or disruptive to other residents and staff. Either way, it is important to determine whether there is a reason for the behavior, and whether the resident needs something.

Kovach (1997) divided repetitive behavior into two types: calm perseverance and tense perseverance. *Calm perseverance* is categorized as calm rhythms of movements or vocalizations that do not tend to escalate. This type of behavior is often a coping mechanism or a response to boredom. *Tense perseverance,* in contrast, is categorized by tense movements or vocalizations that often tend to escalate. Tense behaviors are often associated with pain or discomfort. Therefore, some residents may engage in repetitive behavior because they are bored, whereas for others tense behaviors may be a coping mechanism for something, such as being overstimulated in their situation or environment. Still others may be trying to express pain or discomfort. Interventions that staff can try with residents who exhibit repetitive behaviors are listed in "What Staff Can Do."

WHAT STAFF CAN DO

Disruptive Vocalizations

Vocally disruptive behaviors present a problem not only because they indicate that the resident has an unaddressed feeling or need but also because they can be upsetting and disruptive to other residents, visitors, and staff. This section offers some interventions that may minimize these behaviors. Many of these interventions are intended to have a calming effect on the resident, because vocally disruptive behavior is often an expression of agitation. The interventions are organized to address the specific causes of vocally disruptive behavior listed in Table 6.1.

Over- and Understimulation

Excess or competing noises are one of the main causes of overstimulation. When a vocally disruptive resident is in a busy area, take him or her to a quiet place that does not have as many sources of stimulation. Residents who are prone to this behavior may be bothered by the noise and commotion that is associated with large group activities or eating in large, full dining rooms. One-to-one and small group activities are best for these residents. Try to reduce the overall noise level on the unit as a preventive measure. Glare also can be a source of visual overstimulation. Glare on floors can be caused by unfiltered sunlight, highly polished floor surfaces, and certain types of lighting. "What the Environment Can Do" in Chapter 5 offers specific ways to reduce glare.

Whereas in some residents disruptive vocalizations may result from receiving too much stimulation from the environment, in other residents these vocalizations may result from understimulation. Positive sources of stimulation can reduce or prevent this behavior in these residents. When a resident's vocalizations seem to be a bid for attention, try to schedule more one-to-one time with this person. Such residents are likely understimulated because they cannot provide themselves with sources of stimulation as a result of immobility or possibly being in restraints. They may be lonely and trying to connect with someone. One direct care staff member from each shift could make a point of spending 5 or 10 minutes with these residents a couple of times during his or her shift. Volunteers may be able to spend time with the residents reading to them, giving them a manicure, brushing their hair, or just talking to them. Residents who are understimulated may benefit from sitting in high-activity locations, where they can observe what is going on. The ideas listed under "Sensory Impairment" also may be helpful for understimulated residents.

Sensory Impairment

Low-functioning residents also may be unable to move independently to find an appropriate level of stimulation, and may be experiencing sensory deprivation. These residents would likely benefit from positive sensory stimulation. Music programs are one of the most common forms of acoustical stimulation, and these can have a calming effect on some residents. These programs can range from group activities such as piano recitals and listening to big band music to individualized music played just for one resident who is vocally disruptive. Individualized music is the most effective when played through headphones because they block out other background noises. One study found that tapes of environmental white noise, such as recordings of the sounds made by oceans and streams, to be effective in decreasing disruptive behaviors (Burgio, Scilley, Hardin, Hsu, & Yancey, 1996).

Olfactory stimulation is a creative source of stimulation that is often underused in long-term care facilities. Aromatherapy is a wonderful approach to providing positive stimulation to residents. Aromatherapy can be conducted with the use of essential oils, such as lavender or sandalwood, which can calm some agitated or restless people. The oils can be applied to a light bulb, which when turned on, diffuses the aroma around the room. Familiar aromas, such as the smell of baking bread or pies, not only can have a calming effect but also can be a source for reminiscence.

Tactile stimulation is also important to consider. As residents become less mobile, they are less able to find interesting sources of tactile stimulation on their own. These residents may enjoy having something soft to hold, such as a pillow or stuffed animal. The Spinoza Company makes a stuffed bear that, when clutched, will play prerecorded messages. As with a tape recorder, messages can be recorded by a family member and played back to the resident to offer reassurance and comfort. Pet therapy is another source of tactile stimulation. Petting a cat, dog, or rabbit can be soothing for some people. Animals offer unconditional love, which can put a smile on the faces of even the saddest residents or those with the greatest level of cognitive impairment.

Other Causes of Disruptive Vocalizations

Whenever a resident's vocally disruptive behavior seems to be the result of depression or a psychosis such as paranoia or anxiety, it is important to seek a medical or psychological evaluation. The resident may have a treatable condition. In addition, staff should interact with these residents in a reassuring, nonconfrontational manner. Depressed residents may benefit from reminiscence. These residents are also often quite lonely and might appreciate special attention, such as one-to-one visits, manicures, or little gifts (e.g., an unexpected snack, a favor or prize from activity supplies, artwork). Residents who moan frequently may be expressing pain. It is important to obtain a medical evaluation to determine whether the resident has any treatable sources of pain. Immobile residents may experience pain when they are not repositioned frequently enough.

When vocally disruptive behavior occurs in conjunction with staff's attempts to help a resident, it is likely that the resident does not understand what staff are trying to do. Specific suggestions for approaching residents are listed in "What Staff Can Do" in Chapter 5. If this appears to be the cause of disruptive vocalizations in some residents, then consider consistently assigning one caregiver from each shift to these residents so that they can become familiar with their caregivers.

The changes in the brain that occur with dementia often cause lowered inhibitions. Residents are no longer aware of the distinction between behaviors that they once considered socially appropriate or inappropriate. Lowered inhibitions in residents with dementia may be expressed as swearing or other foul language. Little can be done to prevent this behavior. Residents may not even be aware that they are using inappropriate language. If residents seem to be using this language in response to something, then it should be considered verbally combative behavior (see Chapter 5 for interventions). In general, it is not appropriate to scold adults for swearing or using foul language. Scolding is degrading, and, unlike children, older adults with dementia are unlikely to learn from the scolding and remember not to repeat the behavior. The only time that scolding may be effective (temporarily) and appropriate is when you can ask the resident to not use those words because children or ladies are in the room. The best solution is to remove the resident from the presence of others for a while, so that other residents are not upset.

Sexual Behaviors

As mentioned previously, a facility may need to manage three broad categories of sexual behaviors. The first relates to sexual intimacy between residents and their nonresident partners. The second is intimacy and sexual relationships between residents that are complicated by whether either resident is married, has dementia, or both. The final issue deals with activities that typically are referred to as inappropriate sexual behaviors. Strategies for interventions vary within each category. However, before addressing the categories of behaviors, a general discussion about facility protocol and policies regarding sexual behaviors and staff training in how to address them is necessary.

Facility Protocol

Resident sexual behavior is a complex issue and usually needs to be addressed on a case-by-case basis. However, outlining some general policies (e.g., providing residents with spouses a private room one night a week, arranging home visits) gives staff, residents, and families an understanding of how issues will be handled as they arise. Issues to consider include

- How residents may have privacy with visitors
- How to determine the informed consent of a resident with dementia
- How to respond to the formation of relationships between residents
- How to respond to residents who are masturbating

The latter portion of this section, which focuses on intervention, provides ideas for possible policies and procedures.

As policies are formed, it is important to share them with all staff members and to make them a part of training for new staff. It is also important to discuss policies with new residents and their families. However, these issues can be uncomfortable for residents and their families to discuss, and thus should be handled delicately. Research findings regarding the attitudes of older adults toward sexuality suggest that many older adults are uncomfortable discussing it (Walker & Ephross, 1999). Likewise, family members may have varying degrees of comfort talking about the sexuality and sexual behaviors of their loved ones. Nevertheless, it is still important to address these issues, although careful consideration should be given when deciding what policies should be discussed. For example, if a married individual is moving into the facility, then it is important to discuss his or her right to privacy and how the facility might accommodate it. The couple may not know what to expect and may be uncomfortable bringing up this private matter for discussion. If a widowed individual with dementia is moving in, then you may want to ask his or her children if they wish to be contacted if their parent expresses interest in, or becomes involved with, another resident. Policies regarding masturbation or inappropriate sexual advances may be brought up only if or when the behaviors become an issue. Each facility must decide what type of approach it would like to take.

Staff Training and Discussion

Staff also experience varying degrees of comfort discussing and addressing sexuality and sexual behaviors. The facility should provide staff with general training that addresses some of the issues discussed in this section, such as the normalcy of older adults desiring and engaging in sexual activity. It also may be helpful to address how people have different viewpoints and the importance of always treating residents in an unbiased manner. For example, some staff may feel homosexuality or masturbation is immoral or inappropriate. It is important for staff to remember not to let these feelings interfere with the care they provide or the attitudes they have toward residents. In addition, staff may have concerns for residents who become involved with other residents (e.g., Is she being taken advantage of? Will his wife be hurt if she sees him holding hands with another resident?). Staff need to be able to talk to someone, such as their supervisor, about their concerns and feelings. However, they should be careful to not gossip among themselves about residents' sexual and intimate relationships. Bauer (1999) stated that, although discussion of residents' day-to-day activities is generally accepted and part of the caregiver role, staff should be aware of residents' rights to privacy and dignity. Staff should consider whether information that they possess is necessary for the caregiving role, as opposed to mere gossip, before passing it on to other staff members.

Intimacy Between a Resident and a Nonresident

Many residents have a spouse or significant other who does not live in the facility. In this situation, it may be helpful to address proactively the issue of privacy at the time of admission. Staff should discuss with the couple how privacy can be provided for them. Some facilities offer a special visiting room for these purposes, while others try to schedule time alone for the couple in the resident's bedroom. Other facilities prefer that the resident go home periodically if intimacy is still desired, although this is sometimes not possible. One facility considered providing a room at a nearby hotel. It is important to keep in mind, though, that sex is not the only reason a couple may want privacy. Many couples appreciate privacy for other forms of intimacy, such as holding hands, kissing, and having private conversations. Determine how your facility can provide privacy, and try to work with the couple to find solutions that appeal to both you and the couple.

Intimacy Between Two Residents

A different set of issues must be considered when two residents who are not married to each other wish to become intimate. If they are both mentally competent, not married, and consenting to the relationship, then the facility probably has no right to try to keep this couple apart. However, if one or both of the residents have spouses, or if one or both have dementia, the facility's position is not as clear cut. If one or both residents have dementia, it is important to determine whether informed consent has been established. The three conditions of informed consent include voluntary participation, mental competence, and awareness of risks and benefits (Lichtenberg & Strzepek, 1990). Lichtenberg and Strzepek also referred to decisions that are based on authentic autonomy. Collopy (1988) defined *authentic autonomy* as decisions that are reflective of the person's character and in keeping with his or her past morals and ethics. Establishing informed consent helps rule out the possibility of one resident being coerced or taken advantage of by another. Lichtenberg and Strzepek (1990) developed a short questionnaire that can be used to determine a person's awareness of the relationship, such as whether he or she is aware of who is initiating the sexual contact, has the ability to avoid exploitation, and has an awareness of the potential risks. In a later publication, Lichtenberg (1997) discussed using a cutoff score of 14 on the Mini-Mental State Examination (MMSE) to determine whether the person should be assessed for his or her competence to participate in an intimate relationship. Residents with scores of 13 or lower are considered unable to consent. This system worked at Lichtenberg's facility but may or may not be appropriate at others, so you should refer to the original sources before deciding to use an MMSE score as an indicator.

If both residents are consenting but one or both are married, then the spouse(s) should be informed of the situation. Ideally, this initial conversation should take place early in the development of the friendship before it reaches what some staff refer to as a "crisis point." Determine how the spouse feels about the developing friendship, both in its early stages and as it progresses (potentially) into something more intimate. Be sure to focus not only on the feelings of the nonresident spouse or the adult children but also on the feelings of the residents involved and what they appear to want. It is often a good idea to bring a minister, a rabbi, or an ethicist from a local university into these conversations. As these conversations progress, you might want to develop a checklist of issues to consider.

After determining the presence or absence of informed consent and determining the spouses'/families' wishes, facility administration may decide not to allow the relationship forming between two residents to develop into a more intimate relationship. When this is the case, facility staff must work hard to try to keep these residents apart. If the attachment has become strong, then they will probably seek each other out on a regular basis. It will be especially important to find a broad range of activities that each individual likes. Encourage them to attend group activities, although not the same ones, and ask staff or volunteers to engage them in activities (e.g., games, reading) as well. Keeping these residents busy, at least initially, likely will prevent them from seeking each other out as much. When this does not work, as a last resort one of the residents can be moved to a different hall or unit if this is feasible.

If some of the involved parties do not want the relationship to continue (e.g., spouse, adult children) but others do (e.g., the involved couple), then you may need to negotiate with the family about what the facility is willing or able to do. It may not be feasible to guarantee that the two residents absolutely can be kept apart at all times. Develop a plan that reasonably reflects what staff can do. This might include assigning additional staff time for activities, finding a volunteer(s) to spend time with the resident(s), or both. If one of the families is still dissatisfied, then they may choose to find another facility for their relative.

Sexually Inappropriate Behaviors

As mentioned previously, sexually inappropriate behaviors typically include masturbating, disrobing in public, touching or grabbing at others, and making verbal advances toward others. Often, the reason these behaviors are considered inappropriate is because they occur in public areas. Engaging in these behaviors in public often is related to a loss of inhibitions and the ability to know what is generally accepted as *appropriate public behavior.* The introduction to this chapter discussed possible reasons for these behaviors as well as why these behaviors may or may not be truly inappropriate. This section addresses possible strategies for dealing with these behaviors.

Masturbation

Masturbation in public almost always needs to be discouraged. The question is, should masturbation in private be discouraged or allowed? As mentioned, it is important to make sure that no medical condition (e.g., urinary tract infection, scabies) contributes to this behavior. Next, staff need to assess whether anyone is bothered by the behavior (e.g., roommate, residents walking by the room). Finally, staff need to consider the needs and rights of the resident. Does masturbating allow the resident an outlet for sexual expression or ease his or her anxiety? If so, engaging in the behavior may be beneficial to the resident's well-being. It is often possible to allow this behavior without upsetting others. When the resident begins to masturbate in public, tactfully redirect him or her back to the bedroom. Close the door or curtain and encourage the resident to continue in private.

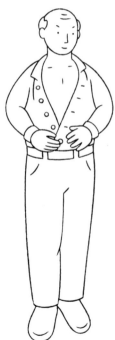

If the resident shares the room with another resident, then make sure the curtain is closed and the other resident is not bothered. It may be necessary to redirect the resident until he or she can be alone in the room.

When masturbating is a recurrent behavior for a resident, staff should track it to determine how often and under what circumstances it occurs. Something in the environment (physical or social) may trigger the behavior. For instance, does Ralph masturbate when he is around women in bathrobes and nightclothes, when soap operas are on television, or when he is in an activity room late in the afternoon and there is no activity going on? To redirect or prevent the behavior, try to determine some of these triggers and make appropriate changes to the environment and program. Eliminate the soap operas, which often are quite explicit in showing sexual activities and behaviors, or develop an activity for the late afternoon. Often, simply finding something for the resident to hold onto can keep his or her hands occupied. Find activities to engage the person; masturbation may be caused by boredom. If masturbating seems to be a positive experience for the resident and the facility decides to allow it in private, then redirect the resident to his or her room and encourage him or her to stay there until finished.

The importance of how staff react to masturbation cannot be emphasized enough. Staff must not overreact or scold the resident in a condescending or judging manner. Rather, staff should quietly approach the resident and ask whether he or she would like to return to the bedroom for a little privacy. If the resident does not want to leave, and the behavior is disturbing others, gently try to remind the resident that some behaviors typically are not done in public. Sometimes using a line such as "there are ladies present" can be effective. Keep in mind that some residents may be experiencing the lack of a sexual partner for the first time in years, and they must find new ways to deal with their sexual needs.

Sexual Advances

Residents who make sexual advances toward staff or other residents may not be after sex but emotional intimacy with another person. A resident with dementia may not be able to articulate this need or desire clearly and as a result may engage in behaviors that are perceived as inappropriate. Residents who frequently touch others simply may be looking for positive affection. Staff can provide appropriate touching in a variety of ways that may help the resident feel an emotional connection with them. Appropriate touch can include holding the resident's hand, resting a hand on the resident's arm while talking with him or her, and hugging. These types of touch convey a caring attitude and may help fulfill residents' needs for intimacy. Including foot massages and back rubs as a regular part of the activity program also provides residents with positive human contact, which is a basic human need.

Disrobing and Exposing Oneself

The text at the beginning of the chapter explained that residents who disrobe in public or expose themselves as a result of unfastened clothing often do not have a sexual motive. Therefore, staff must determine what is causing the behavior: Is the resident hot? Does he or she need to go to the bathroom? Did the resident just come from the bathroom and simply forget to zip his or her zipper? Are the buttons on her blouse too small for her to manage? In many cases, determining the cause of the behavior leads to a simple solution. It is important to remember that cognitive deficits as well as impaired finger sensation or dexterity may make it hard for some residents to fasten some articles of clothing. Larger buttons usually are easier to manage. Replacing zippers with Velcro may be helpful in some cases. In most cases, though, it is important for staff to approach the resident who is disrobing or exposing him- or herself in a tactful and caring manner. They should redirect the resident to a private location to assist him or her in fastening or changing clothes so that the attention of other residents is minimized.

Repetitive Behaviors

The following interventions can be tried when residents engage in repetitive movements or vocalizations:

- When residents engage in repetitive movement, make sure that these movements do not abrade skin or cause harm to themselves or others.
- Determine whether the resident is in pain or feels discomfort and treat accordingly.
- If the resident seems bored, then try to interest him or her in an activity or conversation.
- If the environment seems to be too stressful or overstimulating to a resident, then try taking the individual to a quiet, calm place and see if that alleviates the behavior.
- If the resident is disruptive to other residents or to an ongoing program but the behavior is not in any other way harmful, then try to move the individual away from the residents who are becoming disturbed or agitated.

◆ ◆ ◆

A summary sheet follows, which condenses the chapter text into a quick overview. The authors have also provided an area for you to make your own notes about your own staff and facility. Managerial staff may wish to use the summary sheets as handouts to accompany direct care staff training, or to post them by the time clock or nurses' station or include them in staff's pay envelopes.

SOCIALLY INAPPROPRIATE BEHAVIORS
SUMMARY SHEET

1. Disruptive vocalization refers to noises made by residents either intermittently or continuously with or without an understood purpose.

2. Usually, some underlying reason exists for disruptive vocalization such as a need for attention or an expression of pain.
   - Constant crying out for help may be a sign of anxiety, loneliness, or depression, which indicates that a resident is in need of attention or assistance.
   - Constant moaning may indicate undiagnosed pain. Tell the charge nurse when a resident is moaning, so a medical evaluation can be conducted. Often, these sources of pain are treatable.
   - Repetitive use of words may indicate a sensory impairment or a need for sensory stimulation.
   - If the resident is immobile, he or she may need to be moved more frequently. These vocal expressions should not be ignored as a part of the dementing disease, nor should they be viewed as expressions of someone who is extremely demanding.

   Look for ways to comfort residents or respond to their needs.

3. People with dementia often exhibit repetitive behaviors, which may be expressed by either movements or vocalizations. The causes of repetitive behaviors are varied and are similar to disruptive vocalizations. Try to understand the causes of these behaviors and address the residents' needs. Look for ways to reduce their stress levels.

4. It is normal for older adults to still have sexual feelings. Rather than ignoring sexual behaviors, ask your administrator if the facility has a policy related to such behaviors.

5. Staff may have a variety of reactions/feelings about residents' sexuality. Residents may view themselves as being the same age as staff members and have sexual feelings toward them, which may make staff uncomfortable. Discuss what you are experiencing with other staff members or your supervisor and solve problems together.

6. The underlying cause of some sexual behavior is not sexual. For example:
   - A resident may simply have a need for affection or the touch of another person. The activity probably will never go beyond a simple hug or holding hands.
   - Residents who undress in public may be expressing that they are feeling warm or need to use the bathroom. Some residents with dementia may not recognize the difference between a public and a private setting and begin to disrobe. Residents with dementia often exhibit a loss of inhibition. They may also experience disorientation to time or place. These aspects of the disease can lead to the commission of socially inappropriate behaviors.

What Staff Can Do

1. Unintelligible chatter is some residents' only way of expressing discomfort when overstimulated by the environment. Everyone should do his or her part to make the atmosphere on the unit less stressful. For example,
   - Avoid calling out to other staff members
   - Turn down loud music or television programs.
   - Turn off call bells and alarms quickly.
   - Avoid using the public address system if possible, but if you must use it, lower the volume.

YOUR NOTES

Bibliography

Algase, D. (1992a). A century of progress: Today's strategies for responding to wandering behavior. *Journal of Gerontological Nursing, 18*(11), 28–34.

Algase, D. (1992b). Cognitive discriminants of wandering among nursing home residents. *Nursing Research, 41*(2), 78–81.

Anthony, J.S. (1991). Wandering behavior in long-term care. In M.S. Harper (Ed.), *Management and care of the elderly: Psychosocial perspectives* (pp. 175–179). Newbury Park, CA: Sage Publications.

Bauer, M. (1999). Their only privacy is between their sheets. *Journal of Gerontological Nursing, 25*(8), 37–41.

Bridges-Parlet, S., Knopman, D., & Thompson, T. (1994). A descriptive study of physically aggressive behavior in dementia by direct observation. *Journal of the American Geriatrics Society, 42*(2), 192–197.

Bua, R.N. (1997). *The inside guide to America's nursing homes: Ranking and ratings for every nursing home in the United States.* New York: Warner Books.

Burgio, L., Scilley, K., Hardin, M., Hsu, C., & Yancey, J. (1996). Environmental "white noise": An intervention for verbally agitated nursing home residents. *Journal of Gerontology: Psychological Sciences, 51B*(6), P364–P373.

Chou, K., Kaas, M.J., & Richie, M.F. (1996). Assaultive behavior in geriatric patients. *Journal of Gerontological Nursing, 22*(11), 30–38.

Clark, M.E., Lipe, A.W., & Bilbrey, M. (1998). Use of music to decrease aggressive behaviors in people with dementia. *Journal of Gerontological Nursing, 24*(7), 10–17.

Cohen-Mansfield, J., & Werner, P. (1995). Environmental influences on agitation: An integrative summary of an observational study. *American Journal of Alzheimer's Care and Related Disorders & Research, 10*(1), 32–39.

Cohen-Mansfield, J., Werner, P., & Marx, M.S. (1990). Screaming in nursing home residents. *Journal of the American Geriatrics Society, 38,* 785–792.

Collopy, B.J. (1988). Autonomy in long term care: Some crucial distinctions. *Gerontologist, 28*(Suppl.), 10–17.

Dickinson, J., McLain-Kark, J., & Marshall-Baker, A. (1995). The effects of visual barriers on exiting behavior in a dementia unit. *Gerontologist, 35*(1), 127–130.

Evans, L.K. (1991). Nursing care and management of behavioral problems in the elderly. In M.S. Harper (Ed.), *Management and care of the elderly: Psychosocial perspectives* (pp. 191–206). Newbury Park, CA: Sage Publications.

Feldt, K.S., Warne, M.A., & Ryden, M.B. (1998). Examining pain in aggressive cognitively impaired older adults. *Journal of Gerontological Nursing, 24*(11), 14–22.

Gold, M.F. (1996). Creating harmony from discord: Strategies for calming residents with dementia. *Provider, 22*(3), 66–74.

Gwyther, L. (1985). *Care of Alzheimer's patients: A manual for nursing home staff.* Washington, DC: American Health Care Association and the Alzheimer's Disease and Related Disorders Association.

Hall, G., & Buckwalter, K. (1987). Progressively lowered stress threshold: A conceptual model for care of adults with Alzheimer's disease. *Archives of Psychiatric Nursing, 1*(6), 399–406.

Hellen, C.R. (1995). Intimacy: Nursing home resident issues and staff training. *American Journal of Alzheimer's Disease, 10*(2), 12–17.

Hiatt-Snyder, L., Rupprecht, P., Pyrek, J., Brekhus, S., & Moss, T. (1978). Wandering. *Gerontologist, 18*(3), 272–280.

Hoeffer, B., Rader, J., McKenzie, D., Lavelle, M., & Stewart, B. (1997). Reducing aggressive behavior during bathing cognitively impaired nursing home residents. *Journal of Gerontological Nursing, 23*(5), 16–23.

Hutchinson, S., Leger-Krall, S., & Wilson, H.S. (1996). Toileting: A biobehavioral challenge in Alzheimer's dementia care. *Journal of Gerontological Nursing, 22*(10), 18–27.

Johnson, D. (1995). Restraint-free care. *Nursing Homes, 44*(8), 26–30.

Kovach, C. (1997). *Late-stage dementia care: A basic guide.* Washington, DC: Taylor & Francis.

Lichtenberg, P. (1997). Clinical perspectives on sexual issues in nursing homes. *Topics in Geriatric Rehabilitation: 12*(4), 1–10.

Lichtenberg, P.A., & Strzepek, D.M. (1990). Assessments of institutionalized dementia patients' competencies to participate in intimate relationships. *Gerontologist, 30*(1), 117–120.

Martino-Saltzman, D., Blasch, B., Morris, R., & Wynn McNeal, L. (1991). Travel behavior of nursing home residents perceived as wanderers and nonwanderers. *Gerontologist, 31*(5), 666–672.

Matteson, M.A., & Linton, A. (1996). Wandering behaviors of institutionalized persons with dementia. *Journal of Gerontological Nursing, 22*(9), 39–46.

McIntosh, L., & Richardson, D. (1994). 30-minute evaluation of incontinence in the older woman. *Geriatrics, 49*(2), 35–43.

Monahan, D.J. (1993). Staff perceptions of behavioral problems in nursing home residents with dementia: The role of training. *Educational Gerontology, 19,* 683–694.

Monsour, N., & Robb, S. (1982). Wandering behavior in old age: A psychosocial study. *Social Work, 27*(5), 411–415.

Namazi, K.H., & Johnson, B.D. (1992). Pertinent autonomy for residents with dementias: Modification of the physical environment to enhance autonomy. *American Journal of Alzheimer's Disease and Related Disorders & Research, 7*(1), 16–21.

Namazi, K., & Johnson, B.D. (1996). Issues related to behavior and the physical environment: Bathing cognitively impaired patients. *Geriatric Nursing, 17*(5), 234–239.

Nissenboim, S., & Vroman, C. (1997). *The positive interactions program of activities for people with Alzheimer's disease.* Baltimore: Health Professions Press.

Omnibus Budget Reconciliation Act of 1987, PL 100-203, §§ 2, 101 Stat. 1330.

Philo, S.W., Richie, M.F., & Kaas, M.J. (1996). Inappropriate sexual behavior. *Journal of Gerontological Nursing, 22*(11), 17–22.

Potts, H.W., Richie, M.F., & Kaas, M.J. (1996). Resistance to care. *Journal of Gerontological Nursing, 22*(11), 11–16.

Rader, J. (1987). A comprehensive staff approach to problem wandering. *Gerontologist, 27*(6), 756–760.

Rader, J., Doan, J., & Schwab, M. (1985). How to decrease wandering: A form of agenda behavior. *Geriatric Nursing, 6*(4), 196–199.

Ryan, D.P., Tainsh, S., Kolodny, V., Lendrum, B., & Fisher, R. (1988). Noise-making amongst the elderly in long term care. *Gerontologist, 28*(3), 369–371.

Ryden, M.B., Feldt, K.S., Oh, H.L., Brand, K., Warne, M.E., Weber, E., Nelson, J., & Gross, C. (1999). Relationships between aggressive behavior in cognitively impaired nursing home residents and use of restraints, psychoactive drugs, and secured units. *Archives of Psychiatric Nursing, 13*(4), 170–178.

Sloane, P. (1996, July 14–17). *Managing the patient with disruptive vocalization.* Paper presented at the Alzheimer's Disease Education Conference, Chicago.

Sloane, P., & Mathew, L. (Eds.). (1991). *Dementia units in long-term care.* Baltimore: The Johns Hopkins University Press.

Thomas, W. (1996). *Life worth living: How someone you love can still enjoy life in a nursing home: The Eden Alternative in Action.* Acton, MA: VanderWyk & Burnham.

Walker, B.L., & Ephross, P.H. (1999). Knowledge and attitudes toward sexuality of a group of elderly. *Journal of Gerontological Social Work, 31*(1/2), 85–107.

Whall, A.L., Black, M., Groh, C., Yankou, D., Kupferschmid, B., & Foster, N. (1997). The effect of natural environments upon agitation and aggression in late stage dementia patients. *American Journal of Alzheimer's Disease, 12*(6), 216–220.

White, M., Kaas, M., & Richie, M.F. (1996). Vocally disruptive behavior. *Journal of Gerontological Nursing, 22*(11), 23–29.

Zeiss, A.M., Davies, H.D., & Tinklenberg, J.R. (1996). An observational study of sexual behavior in demented male patients. *Journal of Gerontology: Medical Sciences, 51A*(6), M325–M329.

Zgola, J.M., & Bordillon, G. (2001). *Bon appetit! The joy of dining in long-term care.* Baltimore: Health Professions Press.

Appendix A
Behavior
Tracking
Form

Behavior Tracking Process Form

Behavior being tracked: _____

Who (resident's name)	When (Time it occurred)	Where (Place it occurred)	What		Why (Why do you think the resident behaved this way?)
			(What is the resident doing?)	(What is happening on the unit?)	

Creating Successful Dementia Care Settings, developed by Margaret P. Calkins, Ph.D., M.Arch. © 2002 I.D.E.A.S., Inc.

Behavior Tracking Process Form

Behavior being tracked: _Leaving the unit_

Who (resident's name)	When (Time it occurred)	Where (Place it occurred)	What		Why (Why do you think the resident behaved this way?)
			(What is the resident doing?)	(What is happening on the unit?)	
Calvin T.	9:15 a.m.	By elevator	He followed a visitor onto the elevator	Half of the residents are in activity room for "Coffee Hour"; the rest are in their rooms or by the nurses' station	I think Calvin was just following the visitor—he didn't really want to leave.
Alice B.	11:45 a.m.	Door to stairway in C Wing	She tried to leave through door and set off the alarm	A lot of commotion. Staff are helping residents to dining room. Housekeeping staff are on unit.	I think Alice was overwhelmed by all of the activity on the unit and wanted to get away.
Stanley W.	2:15 p.m.	Main entrance (door unlocked)	He walked out the front door.	Some residents engaged in activity; some napping; about 8 sitting by nurses' station; 5 or 6 wandering	He said something about wanting to check the weather.
Emma S.	3:30 p.m.	Main entrance (door unlocked)	She was trying to leave; I stopped her before she did.	Similar to box above	I asked Emma where she was going. She said she had to get home because her kids would be home from school.

Creating Successful Dementia Care Settings, developed by Margaret P. Calkins, Ph.D., M.Arch. © 2002 I.D.E.A.S., Inc.

Appendix B
Sensory Stimulation Assessment

The environments of some long-term care facilities overstimulate their residents, and the sources of stimulation are not always positive in nature (e.g., acoustic stimulation comes from alarms and call bells instead of pleasant music and conversation). This excess or negative stimulation can influence disruptive behaviors among residents. Consider conducting a sensory stimulation assessment if you believe that some of the disruptive behaviors on your unit may be a result of overstimulation.

The focus of this assessment is to take a closer look at the sources of sound and sights on your unit at various times. The form on page 133 can be used to conduct the assessment. In general, the person who is conducting the assessment should close his or her eyes and listen for 30–60 seconds, and then write down every sound he or she heard during that period. These sounds should include anything heard from people, equipment, public address systems, and the like. Each sound should be recorded in one of the spaces in the left column of the form, and the person should indicate whether he or she thinks the sound is pleasant or unpleasant and how loud it is. Next, the person should look around and record what is happening and how things look at that time. For example, he or she should indicate how many people (i.e., staff and residents) are sitting, how many are moving, and if there are any objects (e.g., carts, empty wheelchairs) that seem abandoned. Always remember to fill in the time of the observation.

There are a few different ways to implement this assessment depending on what problem you are trying to address. If there are recognized periods during which disruptive behaviors occur, then conduct a few assessments just before and during these times. For instance, if you notice a great deal of sundowning on the unit, then try doing an assessment every half hour, beginning 1 hour before the sundowning generally begins and continuing through the period of the disruptive behaviors. However, if you have a problem with noisy, combative, or disruptive behaviors throughout the day, try a different approach. Ask someone from each shift to fill out the assessment 8–12 times during their shift, allowing at least 30 minutes between each assessment. This approach helps provide a picture of how levels and sources of stimulation vary throughout the day.

It is always useful to conduct the assessment from the standpoint of the residents by doing it in places where the residents spend time. For example, complete one assessment seated in the dining room during a meal, another during an activity program, and another sitting among residents who are by the nurses' station or in a day room. This helps you hear and see things from their perspective rather than from your perspective as caregiver.

It is important to remember that, when we are familiar with certain aspects of the environment, they have a tendency to blend into the background. Therefore, consider having multiple people complete one assessment at the same time, and then compare their different observations. A good mix might be a direct care staff member who spends all of his or her time on the unit; an administrative person who only spends a little bit of time on the unit each day; and a nurse, a member of the activity staff, or therapist who spends some of each day on the unit. You might even ask an involved family member to do an assessment. Because people hear and see things differently, use their feedback to highlight to staff that what residents see and hear may be different from what the staff see and hear. People can be educated to be more sensitive to their surroundings.

Once several assessments have been completed, consider the nature of the sounds that staff heard. If many unpleasant noises were heard, can something be done to alleviate any of them? For example, could the use of the public address system be decreased or staff encouraged to respond faster to call bells so that they do not ring continuously. Next, review what staff saw during their observations. Can this information be used to schedule resident and staff activities more effectively? If the assessments find that a lot of staff carts (e.g., linen, medications, housekeeping) are on the unit when residents are not engaged in an activity, consider whether either an activity can be provided for residents at this time or the carts can be brought on the unit at another time.

Sensory Stimulation Assessment

Date observed: _____ Time observed: _____

What you heard	Nature of sound	Level of sound
	❑ Pleasant ❑ Unpleasant ❑ Neutral	❑ Disruptively loud ❑ Loud ❑ Heard above background noise ❑ Part of background noise
	❑ Pleasant ❑ Unpleasant ❑ Neutral	❑ Disruptively loud ❑ Loud ❑ Heard above background noise ❑ Part of background noise
	❑ Pleasant ❑ Unpleasant ❑ Neutral	❑ Disruptively loud ❑ Loud ❑ Heard above background noise ❑ Part of background noise
	❑ Pleasant ❑ Unpleasant ❑ Neutral	❑ Disruptively loud ❑ Loud ❑ Heard above background noise ❑ Part of background noise
	❑ Pleasant ❑ Unpleasant ❑ Neutral	❑ Disruptively loud ❑ Loud ❑ Heard above background noise ❑ Part of background noise
	❑ Pleasant ❑ Unpleasant ❑ Neutral	❑ Disruptively loud ❑ Loud ❑ Heard above background noise ❑ Part of background noise

What you saw (include number of people and what they are doing as well as objects [e.g., carts, empty wheelchairs, holiday decorations])

People: _____

_____

_____

_____

Objects: _____

_____

Creating Successful Dementia Care Settings, developed by
Margaret P. Calkins, Ph.D., M.Arch. © 2002 I.D.E.A.S., Inc.

Sensory Stimulation Assessment

Date observed: _10/22/01_   Time observed: _11:30 a.m._

What you heard	Nature of sound	Level of sound
Sing-along	☒ Pleasant ❑ Unpleasant ❑ Neutral	❑ Disruptively loud ❑ Loud ☒ Heard above background noise ❑ Part of background noise
Call bells	❑ Pleasant ☒ Unpleasant ❑ Neutral	❑ Disruptively loud ❑ Loud ☒ Heard above background noise ❑ Part of background noise
Stan yelling at Emma	❑ Pleasant ☒ Unpleasant ❑ Neutral	☒ Disruptively loud ❑ Loud ❑ Heard above background noise ❑ Part of background noise
Air conditioner	❑ Pleasant ❑ Unpleasant ☒ Neutral	❑ Disruptively loud ❑ Loud ❑ Heard above background noise ☒ Part of background noise
Women talking	☒ Pleasant ❑ Unpleasant ❑ Neutral	❑ Disruptively loud ❑ Loud ☒ Heard above background noise ❑ Part of background noise
Squeaky housekeeping cart	❑ Pleasant ☒ Unpleasant ❑ Neutral	❑ Disruptively loud ☒ Loud ❑ Heard above background noise ❑ Part of background noise

What you saw (include number of people and what they are doing as well as objects [e.g., carts, empty wheelchairs, holiday decorations])

People: _6 residents are sitting by the nurses' station; 8 residents are in the day room watching TV;_

2 housekeepers are in the hall; 3 staff members are behind the nurses' station; 4 residents

are walking around.

Objects: _2 housekeeping carts, 2 med carts, Halloween decorations, 1 lift, birthday balloon bouquet_

on nurses' station counter.

Creating Successful Dementia Care Settings, developed by
Margaret P. Calkins, Ph.D., M.Arch. © 2002 I.D.E.A.S., Inc.

Index

Page numbers followed by *f* indicate figures; those followed by *t* indicate tables. This is a comprehensive index covering Volumes 1–4 of *Creating Successful Dementia Care Settings*. The first number of each entry indicates the volume; the second number indicates the page.